An Atlas of Surgical Approaches to the Bones of the Horse

DENNIS W. MILNE, D.V.M., M.S.

Diplomate, American College of Veterinary Surgeons;
Former Assistant Professor of Surgery, The Ohio
State University Veterinary College, Columbus, Ohio;
Private Practitioner, East Orange, New Jersey

A. SIMON TURNER, B.V.Sc., M.S.

Diplomate, American College of Veterinary Surgeons,
Assistant Professor of Surgery, Department of Clinical
Sciences, College of Veterinary Medicine, Colorado State
University, Fort Collins, Colorado

TEXT AND COVER ILLUSTRATIONS BY BUD KRAMER, B.S., A.M.I.

Senior Medical Illustrator, Learning Resources,
College of Veterinary Medicine, The Ohio State University

1979

W. B. SAUNDERS COMPANY *Philadelphia • London • Toronto*

W. B. Saunders Company: West Washington Square
Philadelphia, PA 19105

1 St. Anne's Road
Eastbourne, East Sussex BN21 3UN, England

1 Goldthorne Avenue
Toronto, Ontario M8Z 5T9, Canada

Library of Congress Cataloging in Publication Data

Milne, Dennis W

Surgical approaches to the bones of the horse.

Bibliography: p.

1. Horses—Surgery. 2. Bones—Surgery. 3. Veterinary surgery. I. Turner, Anthony Simon, joint author. II. Title. [DNLM: 1. Orthopedics. 2. Veterinary medicine. 3. Bone diseases—Veterinary. 4. Horse diseases—Surgery. SF955 M659s]

SF951.M53 636.1′08′97471 78–64718

ISBN 0–7216–6362–1

Surgical Approaches to the Bones of the Horse ISBN 0-7216-6362-1

Last digit is the print number: 9 8 7 6 5 4 3 2 1

DEDICATION

To our loving wives, Joan Laura and Ann Eloise.

Preface

All illustrations in this book were done by Mr. Batvin Kramer. The drawings are all original and are based on dissections performed on cadavers. As the dissections were performed, rough sketches and photographs were made to produce the finished drawings. The principle reference text was the fifth edition of Sisson and Grossman's *The Anatomy of the Domestic Animals,* edited by Robert Getty and published by W. B. Saunders Company, Philadelphia (1975). This book was used for the identification of structures and for the nomenclature in this book. Names of structures that are more commonly used by veterinarian surgeons are also given in the text, in parentheses, beside the correct name.

The authors wish to express their thanks to a number of individuals for their help in making this book possible. We are indebted to Dr. Albert A. Gabel, Professor of Surgery, The Ohio State University College of Veterinary Medicine for the surgical training, direction, and inspiration he gave throughout our surgical residency. Dr. Milne is also grateful to Dr. L. L. Kramer, former Associate Professor of Surgery, Western College of Veterinary Medicine, Canada, for his undergraduate training and to Dr. J. F. Fessler, Professor of Surgery, Purdue University, for his instruction during his surgical internship. We would also like to express appreciation to the Learning Resources Division, College of Veterinary Medicine, The Ohio State University, for allowing us to use their facilities during the dissections.

DENNIS W. MILNE
A. SIMON TURNER

Notes on the Bibliography

The surgical approaches described in this text were referenced when major references were available. These references will give the reader further details about the indications for each approach. The reader is encouraged to read this literature, as it will provide insight into the particular orthopedic procedure associated with the described surgical approach. In some cases, the approach used by the reference authors differs slightly from those described in this text. The approaches described are those preferred by us.

It is not the purpose of this book to discuss orthopedic principles or technical methods for repair, diagnosis, or prognosis. The purpose of this text is to describe the most atraumatic approach to expose a particular bone. Some of these approaches will be used only rarely, such as the approach to the coxofemoral joint in foals. Insufficient numbers of these infrequently used approaches have been recorded in the literature to regard them as "time honored." Other approaches, such as arthrotomy of the carpal joint, have been used successfully by equine surgeons for many years.

Contents

section one

INTRODUCTION

POSITIONING AND PADDING OF THE EQUINE ORTHOPEDIC PATIENT

The correct positioning and adequate padding of the equine orthopedic patient is an essential part of any surgical procedure. The patient must be positioned so the surgeon is not placed in an awkward position, which will lead to early fatigue of the surgeon and will severely compromise technique. Failure to adequately pad and position the horse will result in postoperative problems that can be severe enough to lead to the demise of the animal.

In each approach described in this book, the correct position of the horse has been stated. It is important that the exact location of the lesion be ascertained from radiographs prior to attempting any orthopedic surgery. Human error in marking radiographs is a potential area for mistakes which can lead to incorrect positioning of the patient and failure to find the lesion. This is particularly important in joint surgery in the horse. For example, to approach a chip fracture of the radial carpal bone medial to the extensor carpi radialis tendon, the horse must be in lateral recumbency with the affected limb down. We strongly advise that prior to making the incision, the correct limb and the correct side of the limb be identified. If there is any doubt, surgery should not proceed and properly identified radiographs should be taken.

Complications related to prolonged recumbency of the equine orthopedic patient should be prevented at all costs. Anesthesia of any species is essentially a double-edged sword. While providing analgesia suitable for movement-free surgery, the anesthetized patient can be placed into positions that he would not tolerate when conscious. Anesthetic depression produces muscle relaxation, leading to collapse of the venous return, thereby producing inadequate circulation to affected muscles.

The problems associated with prolonged recumbency are most applicable to adult horses. This includes positional rhabdomyolysis ("tying-up," or azoturia), and radial and peroneal nerve paresis. Especially prone are overweight horses, the larger draught breeds, and athletic horses with fractures. It is the surgeon's responsibility to insure that there is no malpositioning and that the padding is adequate. In lateral recumbency, it is especially important to pull forward and pad the shoulder of the "down" limb.[3] The larger muscle masses of the rear limbs should be padded, and at no stage should any part "overhang" the edge of the table without suitable padding. To improve venous return in the hind limbs while in lateral recumbency, they should be kept abducted, thereby reducing occlusion of the saphenous vein.[1]

Some fractures can be operated on while the animal is in dorsal recumbency. This will eliminate problems associated with pressure on the "down" limbs. It will enable the surgeon to operate on two separate sites without having to take the time to roll the horse and redrape the limb. Draping may be more difficult in dorsal recumbency. Care must be taken to eliminate the hoof from the surgical site to prevent contamination. From the standpoint of adequate ventilation, it has been shown that lateral recumbency is better than dorsal recumbency during general anesthesia.[2]

If limb traction devices are used, they should be used judiciously and be well padded to avoid damage to the nerves and vessels.

References

1. Heath, R. B., Redder, J., Stashak, T. and Shaw, R.: Protecting and Positioning The Equine Surgical Patient. Vet. Med. Small Anim. Clin. November, 1972 1241–1245.
2. Steffey, E. P., Wheat, J. D., Meagher, D. M., Norrie, R. D., McKee, J., Brown, M., and Arnold Jr.:

Body Position and Mode of Ventilation Influences Arterial pH, Oxygen and Carbon Dioxide Tensions in Halothane — Anesthetized Horses. Am. J. Vet. Res. *38*(3) (1977): 370–382.

3. Trim, C. M., and Mason, J.: Post Anesthetic Forelimb Lameness in Horses. Eq. Vet. J. *5*(2): 71–76, April, 1974.
4. Waldron-Mease, E.: Post Operative Muscle Damage in Horses. J. Eq. Med. Surg. *1*(3):106–110, March 1977.

ASEPTIC TECHNIQUE AND STERILIZATION

As well as knowledge of anatomy and physiology, correct and adequate exposure, hemostasis, and atraumatic handling of bone and soft tissues, a good surgeon must have a working knowledge of aseptic technique.

All surgical procedures should be carried out using strict aseptic technique. This is particularly important when entering joints or using metallic implants. Joint infections are difficult to treat and can leave the patient completely debilitated. The combination of infection and instable implants may lead to non-union of fractures with extensive soft tissue damage. This can be particularly devastating in the horse because it may result in disuse and dysfunction of a limb, and thereby limit the animal's ability as an athlete. Good aseptic technique requires more than attention to what transpires in the operating theater. It necessitates an understanding of the principles of instrument sterilization as well.

Sterilization of the surgical instruments and equipment should be done using a steam autoclave (moist heat sterilization) or ethylene oxide (gas sterilization). These are the most common methods of sterilization. Chemical sterilization should not be used. Chemicals, although they are germicidal to some extent, do not kill all spores and the absolute strength of the solution is not always known. Longer periods of time are sometimes required for them to be effective. This is very often impractical.

Sterilization using steam under pressure in an autoclave will kill all spores if the moist heat is in direct contact with every surface of an item. It will, however, dull sharp instruments in time and will damage some surgical instruments that are heat labile. The interior of a surgery pack is most important, and sterilization indicators* should be placed in the middle of the pack at the time of wrapping to insure proper penetration of moist heat. This allows the surgeon to check for adequate sterilization at the time of opening the pack. Commonly used are the color changing indicators. The autoclave must be loaded loosely to allow steam circulation between packages. The recommended temperature for general use in steam sterilization is 250° F (121° C) for 30 minutes. There is usually a 15 minute drying period. Packs should not exceed 12 × 12 × 20 inches in size and should weigh no more than 10 to 12 pounds. The pack must be loosely but securely wrapped. The instruments should be placed in a pattern that will be convenient to the surgeon when they are opened.

Box locks on the instruments should be left open. Some instruments may have to be dismantled for autoclaving. Instruments must be free of oil and grease. All wrapping material must be dry and intact with no holes, tears or stains. Wrapping material should consist of double layer (140 thread count) muslin.

It is recommended that rubber goods be autoclaved for at least 15 minutes at 250° F. Rubber tubing in which the steam only partially displaces the air should be autoclaved for a period of at least 30 minutes (250° F) to compensate for the lower temperature in the tubing. The mechanical cleansing of the tubing prior to sterilization is a factor in the reduction of the bacterial count in its lumen. Some moisture

*Sterilometer, American Hospital Supply, Division of American Hospital Supply Company, McGraw Park, Illinois.

remaining in its lumen will actually turn to steam as the temperature rises and aid in displacing the air in the tubing, thereby increasing the temperature within it.

Packs should be allowed to dry, and warm packs *should not* be placed on cold surfaces, as they become damp owing to condensation and are therefore contaminated.

Ethylene oxide sterilization is used primarily for heat sensitive items but can be used for virtually all instruments. Plastics such as polypropylene, polyethylene rubber goods, endoscopic equipment, and electric cords are not damaged by ethylene oxide sterilization. Ethylene oxide is water soluble at 50° F and is a reliable agent for the destruction of microorganisms. It is usually combined with an inert gas such as Freon or a fluorinated hydrocarbon to reduce the flammability and toxicity of the pure substance. In the process of gas sterilization, temperature, humidity and gas concentration are important. Heat is applied at 100 to 160° F, with a gas concentration of 450 to 1000 mg per liter and a relative humidity of 20 to 40 per cent. The goods are exposed for 1½ to 6 hours (130° for 3 hours is recommended). Goods are usually wrapped in plastic packaging material, which the ethylene oxide will penetrate. Cloth wraps may be used for larger items. Some materials, such as rubber gloves, plastic items and rubber tubing, absorb a certain amount of gas which, if allowed to come into contact with the skin, will cause irritation and vesiccation. Therefore, these articles must be allowed to aerate for 24 hours (seven days for rubber goods and prosthetic materials in direct contact with tissues). Ethylene oxide sensitive chemical indicators should be placed in the pack to check for adequate sterilization.

There should be no compromise with sterility. The surgeon should be sure the necessary conditions have been met and that all factors involved in the sterilization process have been painstakingly observed. Antibiotics may tempt the surgeon to become careless under pretense of emergency. Antibiotics are no substitute for asepsis. They are used in individual cases to control a specific kind of bacteria. Their indiscriminate use is to be condemned in clean elective surgery.

The operating room personnel must maintain the highest standard of sterile technique to protect the patient from the disastrous consequences of infection. The surgeon must adhere to aseptic technique at all times.

The following rules should be observed:

1. Sterile instruments must be kept only on sterile surfaces.
2. Sterile surfaces must not be touched by nonsterile personnel.
3. Hands should be kept above the waist and never folded.
4. Sterile instruments should not fall below the waist of the surgeon.
5. All sterile surfaces should be kept dry.
6. Movement and conversation should be kept to a minimum. The number of persons entering and leaving the operating room should be minimal; this has a significant effect on the numbers of airborne bacteria.
7. Those persons considered part of the operating team should never turn their backs on the sterile field.
8. Exercise care when opening sterile instruments, ensuring that the outside wrapper does not come into contact with either the instrument itself or other sterile surfaces.

Reference

1. Gourley, I. M., and Ettleman, P. S.: The surgical supply area and its procedures. Archives 3(Fall, 1973): 55–59.

PREPARATION OF THE SURGICAL SITE

The initial clipping of the surgical site should be performed in an area other than the operating room (using a number 40 clipper blade). A wide area around the surgical site can be washed to remove the gross contamination (dirt and dander). The horse's shoes can be pulled (or wrapped in protective bandages) to prevent injury during induction of anesthesia. The animal should be groomed thoroughly and wiped over with a damp cloth prior to entering the surgical suite.

Several options exist at this stage regarding preparation of the limb for aseptic surgery. For those operations involving the carpus and below, or the tarsus and below, the limb can be prepared surgically and wrapped in sterile bandages while the horse is standing prior to induction. When the patient has been adjusted on the operating table to the desired position, the bandages may be removed and a sterilized Esmarch bandage and tourniquet applied in an aseptic manner. This method reduces the time between the induction of anesthesia and the beginning of surgery. It does, however, require strict adherence to aseptic technique, especially when applying the Esmarch bandage and tourniquet.

If an Esmarch bandage and tourniquet are not to be used, or if the surgical site obviously makes their use impossible (e.g., upper extremities) then the final skin preparation can be performed soon after general anesthesia has been induced.

The final preparation of the surgical site is controversial, and disagreement exists as to the efficacy of various methods. Clipping is essential. Shaving, although not carried out in many human hospitals, is essential in most locations on the horse owing to the much higher density of hair follicles. An area several inches on either side of the proposed surgical site should be shaved. Shaving the night prior to surgery followed by aseptic preparation of the site has led to blistering of fine-skinned horses, especially when the limb is wrapped and exposed to even the mildest of germicides. This may enhance the risk of infection at the surgery site; therefore, shaving of the surgical site should be done just prior to surgery.

After the surgical site has been shaved, the skin can be cleansed further with a surgical scrub to remove dirt, dander, and the natural layer of sebum on the animal's skin. The surgical scrub should be done in a ritualistic manner, beginning over the proposed surgical site and working in a circular fashion to the periphery. When the periphery is reached, the sponges used should be discarded. The surgical scrub should be nonirritating and must not inhibit healing of the wound. A commonly used surgical scrub is povidone-iodine.* Following each scrub, the surgical site can be rinsed with water or alternated with an effective germicidal compound which is fat soluble (such as 70 per cent ethyl alcohol). The final scrub is with alcohol for three minutes. This is then blotted dry with a sterile towel, and a germicidal solution is sprayed on the skin prior to operating.

If sterile adhesive plastic drapes are to be used, the skin should be allowed to dry following the application of alcohol. The site is then sprayed with a surgical adhesive** and an impervious plastic drape may be applied.† Controversy exists as to whether impervious plastic drapes actually reduce the number of wound infections; however, their use has a number of advantages. They do allow the surgical site and the surrounding landmarks to be visualized. This aids the surgeon in the placement of incision because relevant landmarks are not completely obscured by muslin drapes.

---

*Betadine, Purdue-Frederick Co., Norwalk, Ct.

**Vi-Drape Adhesive, Parke Davis & Company, Parke Davis & Company, Ltd.

†Steri-Drape, 3M Animal Care Products, St. Paul, MN. Barrier Incise Drape, Johnson & Johnson Company, New Brunswick, NJ.

The adhesive plastic drapes work well for small incisions. However, in some of the longer incisions, such as approaches to the long bones, there is a tendency for these drapes to become dislodged along the incision site. This will occur especially if there is excessive manipulation associated with fracture reduction. In these cases the surgeon must use judgment as to whether he will use these particular drapes or suture skin towels to the wound edges.

INSTRUMENTATION*

Use of Retractors

Many of the approaches described in this book are facilitated by adequate retraction of the soft tissues. The correct use of appropriate instruments will provide good retraction and exposure. The surgeon should take great care to protect soft tissue structures, as the integrity of these is often the determining factor in the success or failure of the orthopedic procedure(s).

Retractors can be divided into two basic groups, hand-held and self-retaining. The self-retaining retractors are obviously beneficial for the surgeon who has minimal assistance. Self-retaining retractors include the *Weitlaner retractors* (Fig. 1) and the *Gelpi retractors* (Fig. 2). These retractors can develop only a limited amount of force and are of no value in retracting large muscle bellies such as are found in the approaches to the long bones. They are of most value when used in arthrotomies, such as the approaches to the various carpal bones and the approach to the apex of the proximal sesamoid bone. Their insertion into and removal from joint spaces must be done carefully.

Hand-held retractors are available in various sizes and shapes. Like the self-retaining retractors, they must be carefully placed and inserted into such places as joints with precision and exactness. For arthrotomies, the *Miller-Senn* (Senn) retractors (Fig. 3) may be useful. The sharp rakelike end of this retractor can easily puncture gloves and can be difficult to dislodge from the soft tissues. The smoother end is, however, very useful either in combination with another *Senn* or some other type of retractor.

*Illustrations for the instruments shown on these pages have been supplied by the J. Sklar Manufacturing Company, 38–04 Woodside Avenue, Long Island City N.Y. 11101, and by Orthopedic Equipment Company, Inc., Bourbon, IN 46504.

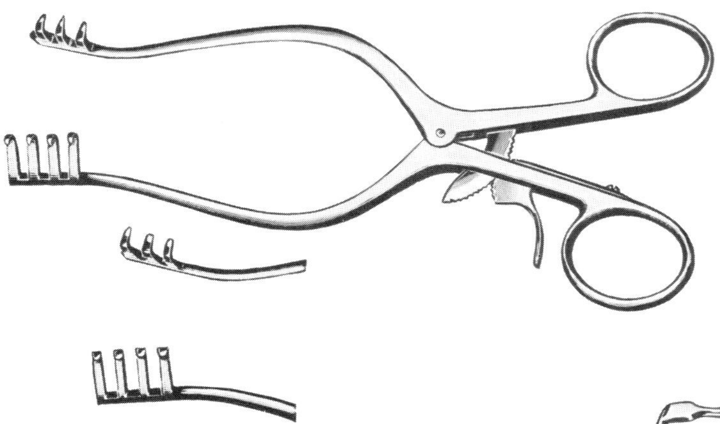

FIGURE 1

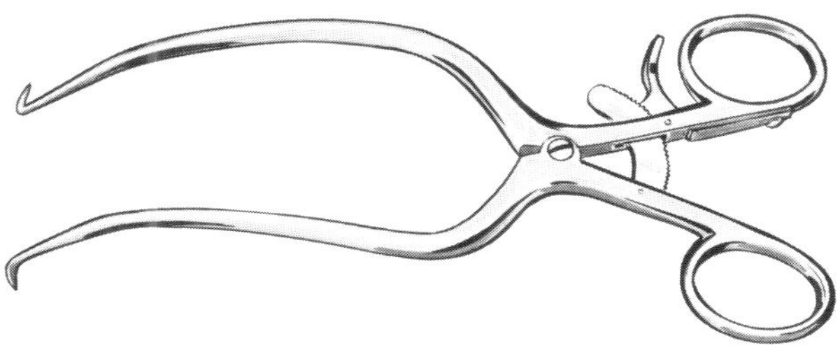

FIGURE 2

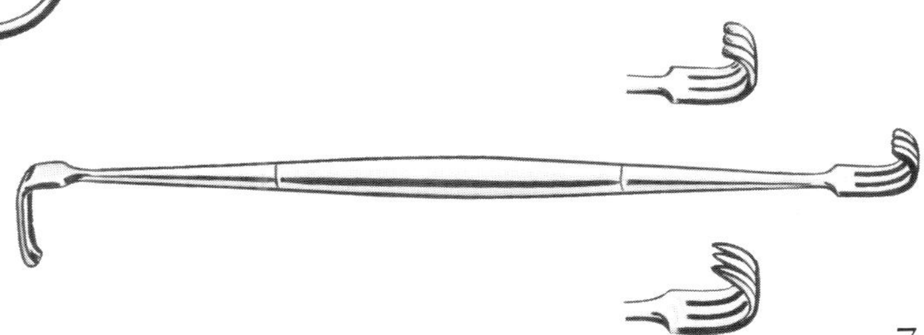

FIGURE 3

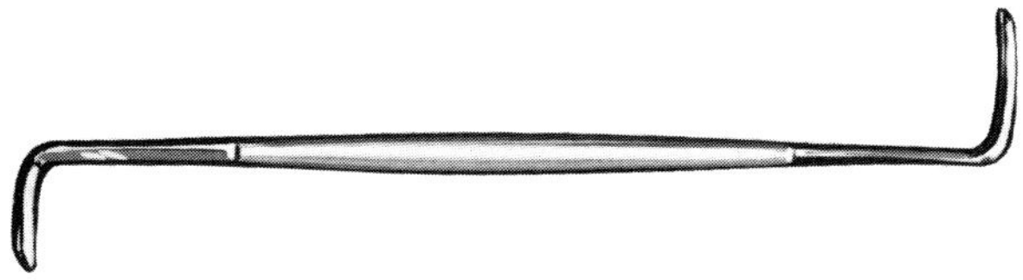

FIGURE 4

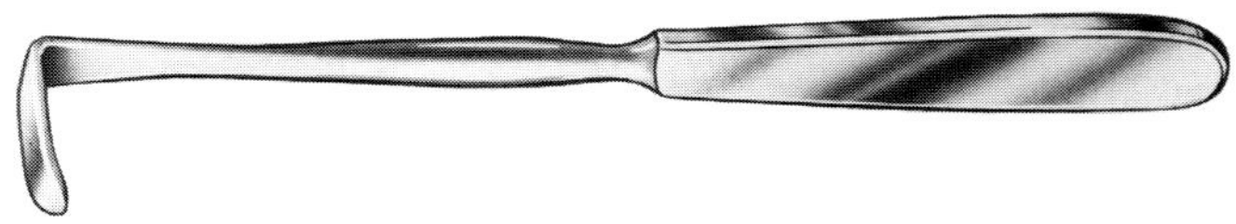

FIGURE 5

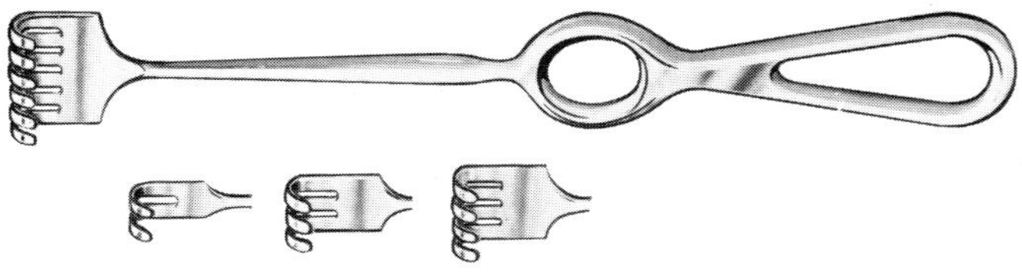

FIGURE 6

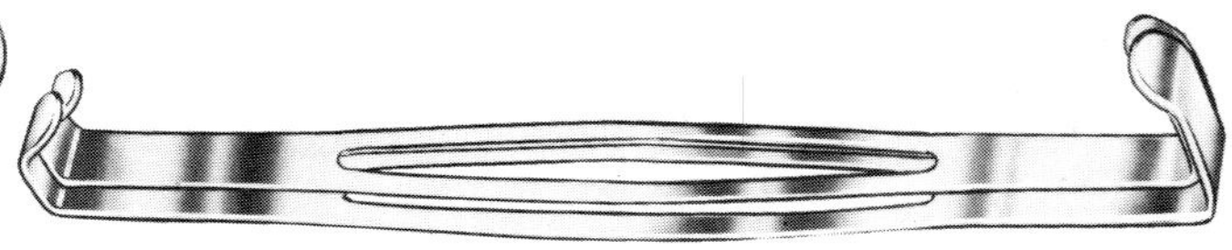

FIGURE 7

Other retractors useful in small incisions such as arthrotomies are the *Davis retractors* (Fig. 4) and *Langenbeck retractors* (Fig. 5). *Volkmann retractors* (Fig. 6) are useful in retracting tendinous structures or joint capsules.

For performing arthrotomies of the carpus, we have found a retractor with a longer wider blade useful for viewing the articular surfaces of the carpal bones under the tendon of the extensor carpi radialis muscle. The longer blade of the *U.S. Army retractor* (Fig. 7) or the blade of a *Sauerbruch retractor* (Fig. 8) is extremely useful for this purpose. To facilitate placement of such a retractor, the carpus is extended fully, relaxing the tendon of the extensor carpi radialis. The blade of the retractor is carefully placed under this tendon, within the joint. The other edge of the joint capsule can be retracted with a retractor of smaller blade width. For retraction of large muscle bellies, U.S. Army retractors and Sauerbruch retractors will be useful.

When the approach results in an incision of some depth *malleable retractors* (Fig. 9) may be useful. However, their use is limited by the amount of pressure that one can develop with them.

For deep dissection, and when considerable muscle tension exists, the various types of *Hohmann retractors* (Fig. 10) are indicated, for example, in the approach to the lateral side of the distal radius for application of a bone plate. To gain access to the anterior surface of the radius, these retractors are useful for retraction of the muscle belly of the extensor carpi radialis.

We have included in instrumentation, the Gigli wire saw (Fig. 11). This is useful for removal of the greater trochanter.

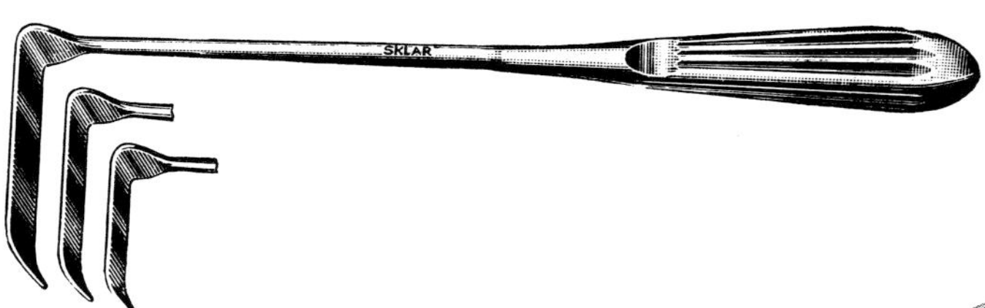

FIGURE 8

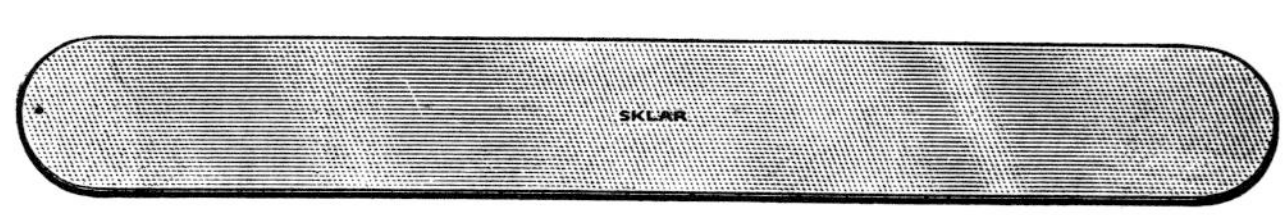

FIGURE 9

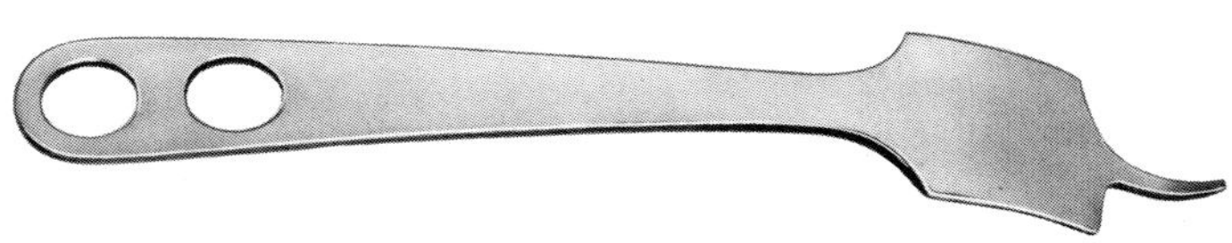

FIGURE 10

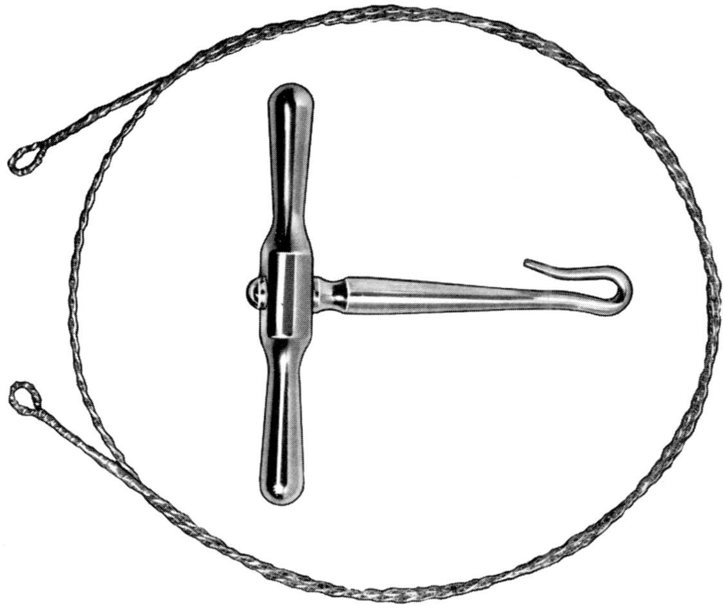

FIGURE 11

SURGICAL APPROACHES TO THE LONG BONES OF THE HORSE*

In 1958, with the development of the Association for the Study of Internal Fixation (ASIF), major advancements were made in the study of internal fixation of fractures. The aim of this group was to design a method of fracture repair that would result in early return to full function without the development of stiff joints and soft tissue damage. Extensive research by this group and others resulted in the conclusion that the desired results for fracture repair could best be obtained by providing rigid internal fixation by using compression techniques. This led to the development of specialized precision instruments.[2, 3, 11, 13, 14]

Although designed for human use, the ASIF equipment has provided a means of successfully treating certain long-bone fractures of the horse.[1, 4-10, 15, 16, 18] In the horse, where immobilization by conservative means is often impossible, internal fixation is important in offering a chance of success. Certain fractures are not amenable to casting. This is particularly true of fractures of the humerus, radius, ulna, femur and tibia, where the joint above the fracture cannot be immobilized, resulting in inadequate stabilization.

Compression techniques with ASIF implants have provided stability and immediate ambulation without external coaptation in the young horse.[16, 18] In the adult horse, the combination of internal fixation with compression plates and external coaptation with casts in carefully selected cases has resulted in successful repair. At present, the combination of compression plate fixation and external coaptation is the most advantageous method of fracture repair in the horse.

Approaches to long bones in the horse are often in areas where only skin and subcutaneous tissue cover the bone. This can pose a problem in closure of the skin over the plate. If the skin incision is straight, it may become superimposed over the plate, resulting in excessive tension on the skin and increased chance of wound

---

*Some of these comments have been extracted from Milne, D. W., *et al*: Surgical Approaches to Certain Long Bones of the Horse for Application of Tension Band Plates. J.A.V.M.A. *168*: 48–52 (January, 1976)

dehiscence. For this reason, curvilinear skin incisions are used for approaches to the radius, ulna, tibia, calcaneus, metacarpus and metatarsus.

Curvilinear skin incisions have their bases over the craniomedial or craniolateral aspect of the fractured bone, thus providing good exposure to the radius, tibia, metacarpus and metatarsus. The apex of the skin incision lies over the soft tissue caudomedial or caudolateral to the bone. The superficial and deep fascia are incised directly over the bone. The skin incision for the approaches to the ulna and calcaneus are made curvilinear only over the olecranon and proximal part of the tuber calcis, respectively, where they are not covered by muscle.

Successful treatment of long-bone fractures, using the ASIF technique, can be accomplished only when the surgeon has a thorough understanding of the ASIF principles, which have been well outlined.[11] It is equally important for the surgeon to have a thorough knowledge of the regional anatomy for the surgical approaches and proper placement of the plates.[12]

The surgical approaches to the long bones described in this text are those most amenable to internal fixation. The bones illustrated and their dimensions for the approaches to the proximal and middle phalanx, metacarpus III, metatarsus III, radius, ulna, tibia, calcaneus, and tuber coxae are of the adult horse. The bones illustrated and their dimensions for the approaches to the humerus, femur, tuber scapulae and dorsal approach to the hip are based on the adolescent (<140 kg.) horse's limb. The surgical approach described for each bone represents the most advantageous plate position, based on the anatomic availability and the tension side of the respective bones. The tension side of some of the bones was determined previously.[17]

References

1. Alexander, J. T., and Rooney, J. R.: The Biomechanics, Surgery and Prognosis of Equine Fractures. *In* Proceedings 18th Annual Meeting, American Association of Equine Practitioners, 1972. 219–235: (1973).
2. Allgower, M., Ehrsam, R., Ganz, R., Matler, P., and Perren, S. M.: Clinical experience with a New Compression Plate — DCP. Acta Orthop. Scand. (Suppl), *125* (1969): 45–63.
3. Allgower, M., Mattler, P., Perren, S. M., and Ruedi, T.: The Dynamic Compression Plate (DCP). Berlin, Germany, Springer Verlag, 1973
4. Dingwall, J. S., Duncan, D. B., and Horney, F. D.: Compression Plating in Large Animal Orthopedics. J.A.V.M.A., *158* (1971): 1651–1657.
5. Fretz, P. B.: Fractured Ulna in the Horse. Canad. Vet. J., *14*: 50–53 (1973).
6. Gertsen, K. E., and Brinker, W. O.: Fracture Repair in Ponies Using Bone Plates. J.A.V.M.A., *154*(1969): 900–905.
7. Gertson, K. E., Monfort, T. N., and Tillotson, P. J.: Fracture Repair in Large Animals. Vet. Med. Small. Anim. Clin., *68*(1973): 782–790.
8. Jenny, J.: ASIF Plate Application in Long Bone Fractures. *In* Proceedings 14th Annual Meeting, American Association of Equine Practitioners, 1968. (1969): 171–173.
9. Jenny, J.: ASIF Technique for Fixation of Fractures in the Horse. *In* Proceedings 14th Annual Meeting, American Association of Equine Practitioners, 1968. (1969): 99–100.
10. Johnson, J. H., and Butler, H. C.: The Tension Band Principle in Fixation of an Equine Ulna Fracture. Vet. Med. Small Anim. Clin. *66*(1971): 552–556.
11. Mueller, M. E., Allgower, M., and Willenegger, H.: Manual of Internal Fixation. Berlin, Germany, Springer Verlag, 1970.
12. Milne, D. W., Turner, A. S., and Gabel, A. A.: Surgical Approaches to Certain Long Bones of the Horse for Application of Tension Band Plates. J.A.V.M.A. *168*:(1976): 48–52.
13. Perren, S. M., Russenberger, M., Steinemann, S., Mueller, M. E., and Allgower, M.: A Dynamic Compression Plate. Acta Orthop. Scand. (Suppl.), *125*(1969): 31–41.
14. Perren, S. M., Allgower, M., Cordey, J., and Russenberger, M.: Development of Compression Plate Techniques for Internal Fixation of Fractures. Prog. Surg. *12*(1973): 152–179.
15. Scott, E. A.: Tension-Band Fixation of Equine Ulna Fractures Using Semi-Tubular Plates *In* Proceedings 21st Annual Meeting, American Association of Equine Practitioners, 1975. (1976): 167–176.
16. Turner, A. S., Milne, D. W., and Gabel, A. A.: The Dynamic Compression Plate in Equine Long Bone Fractures. J.A.V.M.A., *168*(1976): 309–315.
17. Turner, A. S., Mills, E. J., and Gabel, A. A.: In Vivo Measurement of Bone Strain in the Horse. Am. J. Vet. Res., *36*(1975): 1573–1579.
18. Turner, A. S. Surgical Repair of a Fractured Femur in a Foal. J. Equine Med. Surg., *1*(5)(1977): 180–185.

section two

THE THORACIC LIMB

part one

Approach to the Distal Phalanx

CRANIAL APPROACH TO EXTENSOR PROCESS OF DISTAL PHALANX (THIRD PHALANX)

INDICATIONS

1. Removal of avulsion fractures of the extensor process of the distal phalanx.[1, 2, 4]
2. Open reduction and fixation of avulsion fractures of the extensor process.[3, 5]

POSITIONING OF THE PATIENT

The patient is placed in right or left lateral recumbency with the affected limb uppermost.

DESCRIPTION OF PROCEDURE

A. *Topographical View.* A skin incision is made extending from the coronary band to approximately 4 cm. proximally.

B. *Diagrammatic View of Tendons, Ligaments, and Vessels in Relationship to Bones.* The incision is placed over the cranial aspect of the distal interphalangeal joint so that it bisects the common digital extensor tendon.

CRANIAL APPROACH TO EXTENSOR PROCESS OF DISTAL PHALANX (THIRD PHALANX)

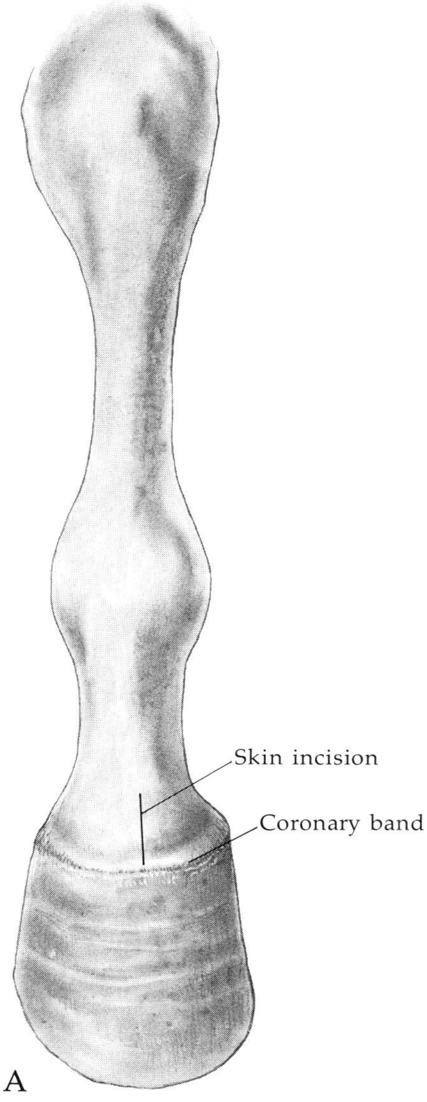

A

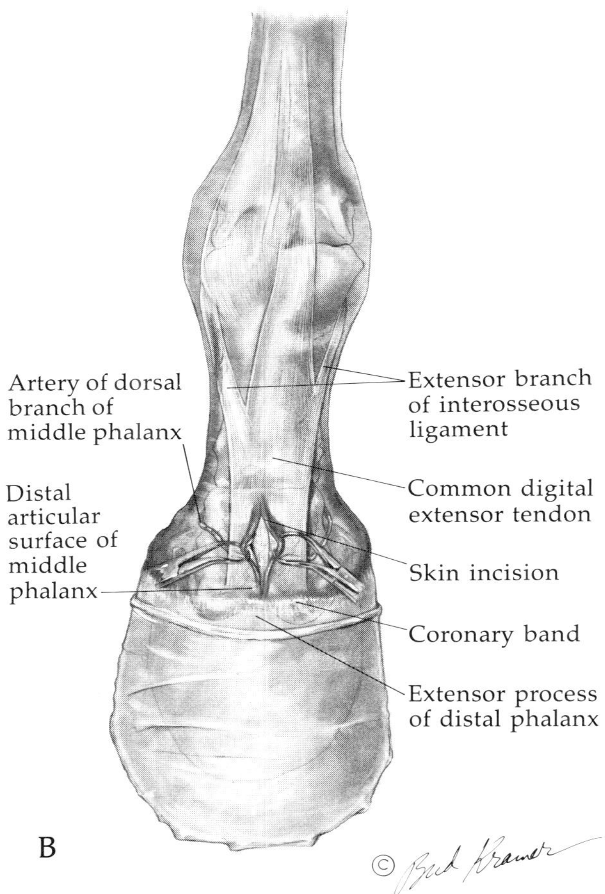

B

C. *Surgeon's View.* The subcutaneous fascia, common digital extensor tendon, and joint capsule are incised along the same line as the skin incision. When making the incision in the joint capsule the artery of the dorsal branch of the middle phalanx should be identified at the proximal extent of the incision. If the incision in the joint capsule needs to be extended to provide further exposure, this vessel may be transected and ligated. The two margins of the joint capsule are retracted laterally and medially as the distal interphalangeal joint is flexed.

D. *Diagrammatic View of Middle and Distal Phalanx.* The extensor process lies distal to the coronary band. Flexing and extending the distal interphalangeal joint will facilitate exposure of the extensor process and articular surfaces.

CLOSURE

Because of the close apposition of the joint capsule to the common digital extensor tendon, closure of the joint capsule as a separate layer can be difficult. It is often necessary to include inner layers of the tendon in the closure of the joint capsule. A simple interrupted pattern is recommended. The outer layers of the common digital extensor tendon should be closed with a simple interrupted suture pattern. A simple or continuous suture pattern can be used in the subcutaneous tissues. The skin is closed using an interrupted suture pattern with the incised edges in firm apposition.

COMMENTS

On completion of the incision into the distal interphalangeal joint, the most apparent bony structure will be the distal articular margin of the middle phalanx. The surgeon should not mistake this for the extensor process of the distal phalanx, which is difficult to see since it lies distal to the most distal end of the incision, deep to the coronary band.

References

1. Adams, O. R.: Lameness in Horses. 3rd ed., Philadelphia, Lea and Febiger, 1974, pp. 241–243.
2. Duncan, D. B., and Dingwall, J. S.: Surgical Removal of Avulsed Portions of the Extensor Process of the Third Phalanx in the Horse. J.A.V.M.A. *159*(1971):201–203.
3. Haynes, P. F., and Adams, O. R.: Internal Fixation of Fractured Extensor Process of Third Phalanx in a Horse. J.A.V.M.A. *164*(1974):61–63.
4. Von Leuthold, A.: Navicular Disease and Fracture of the Extensor Process of the Third Phalanx. Schweiz. Arch. Tierheilkd. *117*(1974):469–473.
5. Petterson, H.: Fractures of the Pedal Bone in the Horse. Equine Vet. J. *8*(1976):104–109.

CRANIAL APPROACH TO EXTENSOR PROCESS OF DISTAL PHALANX (THIRD PHALANX)

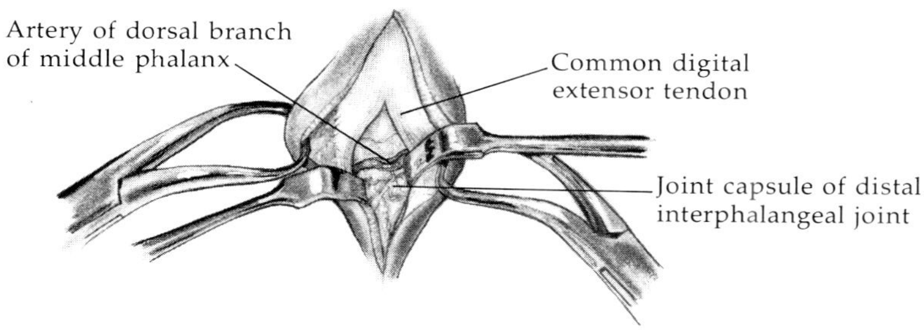

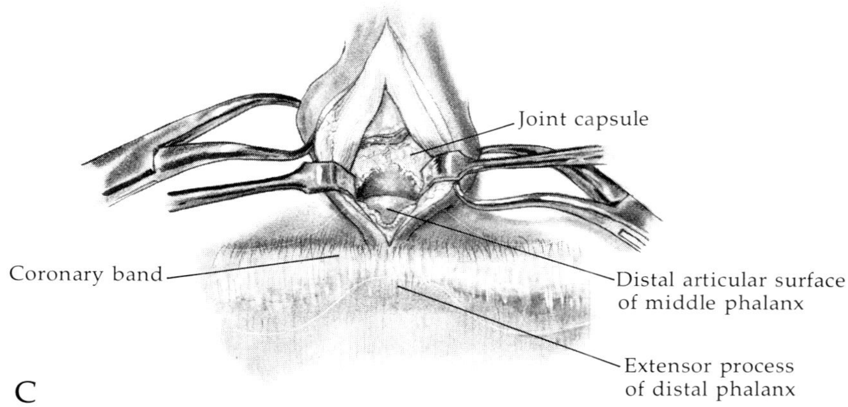

C

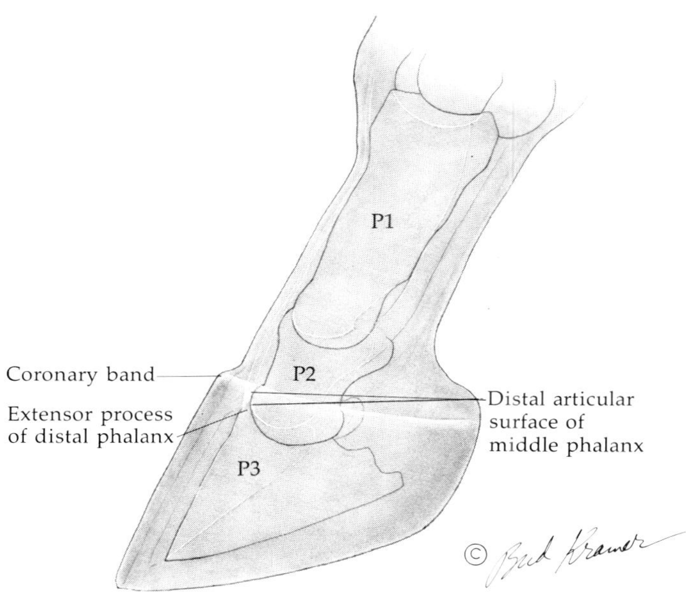

D

part two

Approach to the Proximal Phalanx and Third Metacarpus

CRANIAL APPROACH TO THE PROXIMAL PHALANX AND THIRD METACARPUS (Mc III)

INDICATION

1. Arthrodesis of the fetlock (metacarpophalangeal) joint.

POSITIONING OF THE PATIENT

The horse is positioned in right or left lateral recumbency with the affected limb uppermost.

DESCRIPTION OF PROCEDURE

A. *Topographical View.* An inverted "T"-shaped incision approximately 24 cm. long is made over the cranial surface of the proximal phalanx extending up Mc III to approximately the junction of the middle and proximal third of its cranial shaft. The distal part of the incision is placed across the distal border of the proximal phalanx.

CRANIAL APPROACH TO THE PROXIMAL PHALANX AND THIRD METACARPUS (Mc III)

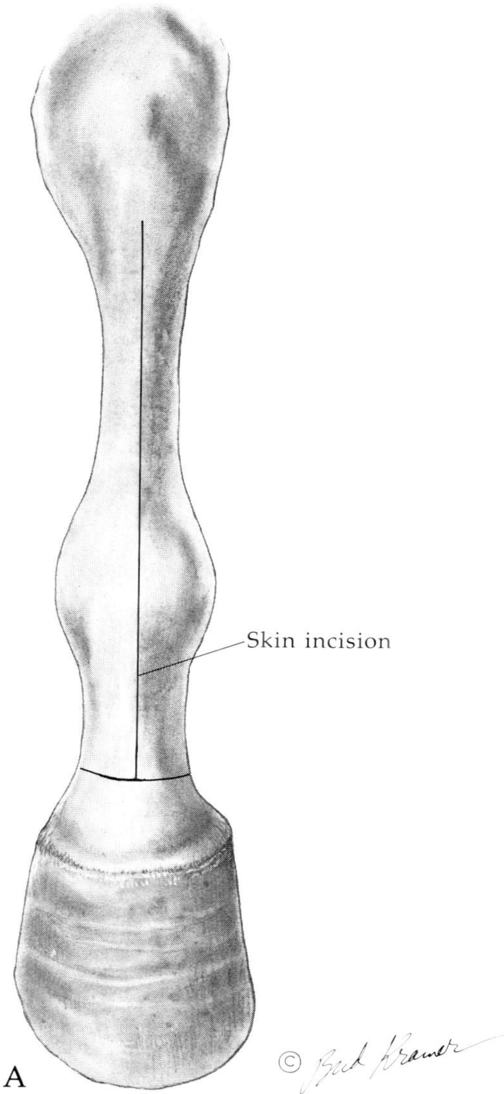

A

CRANIAL APPROACH TO THE PROXIMAL PHALANX AND THIRD METACARPUS (Mc III)

B, C, and D. Surgeon's View. The skin is reflected medially and laterally from the midline, exposing the common digital extensor tendon and the two extensor branches of the interosseous ligament. A Z-plasty is performed in the common digital extensor tendon and the two extensor branches of the interosseous ligament. The tendons are reflected from the cranial surface of the first phalanx and Mc III. This exposes the underlying bone and fetlock joint capsule.

CLOSURE

The incisions in the tendons are reapposed using a simple interrupted pattern with a nonabsorbable suture material. The skin should be closed with an interrupted suture pattern with the incised edges in firm apposition.

COMMENTS

The skin on the cranial surface of the first phalanx lacks mobility. Placing metal implants on the cranial surface of the first phalanx beneath this nonmobile skin predisposes to postoperative wound dehiscence. Therefore, during surgery, the surgeon must be very meticulous in protecting the skin flaps from inadvertent trauma which may further predispose to postoperative wound dehiscence. To expose the fetlock joint for arthrodesis, the joint is opened transversely and placed in flexion. To adequately expose the articular surfaces of the fetlock joint the medial and lateral collateral ligaments may be partially severed transversely.

CRANIAL APPROACH TO THE PROXIMAL PHALANX AND THIRD METACARPUS (Mc III)

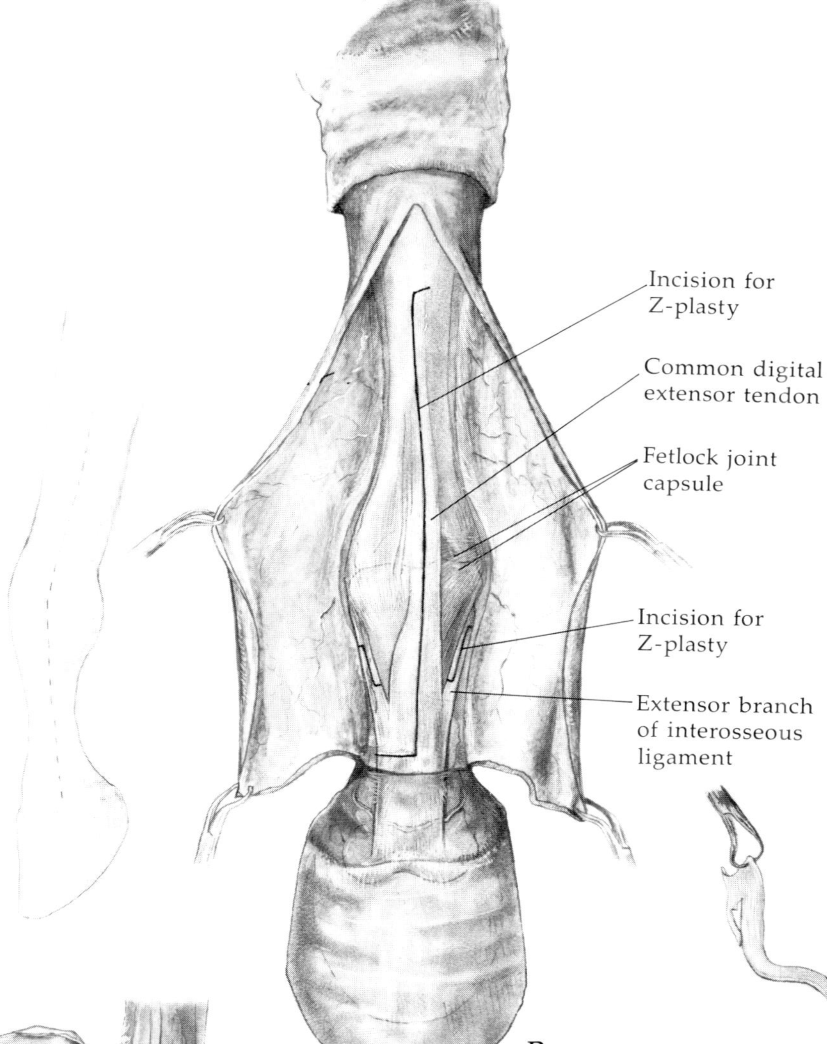

B

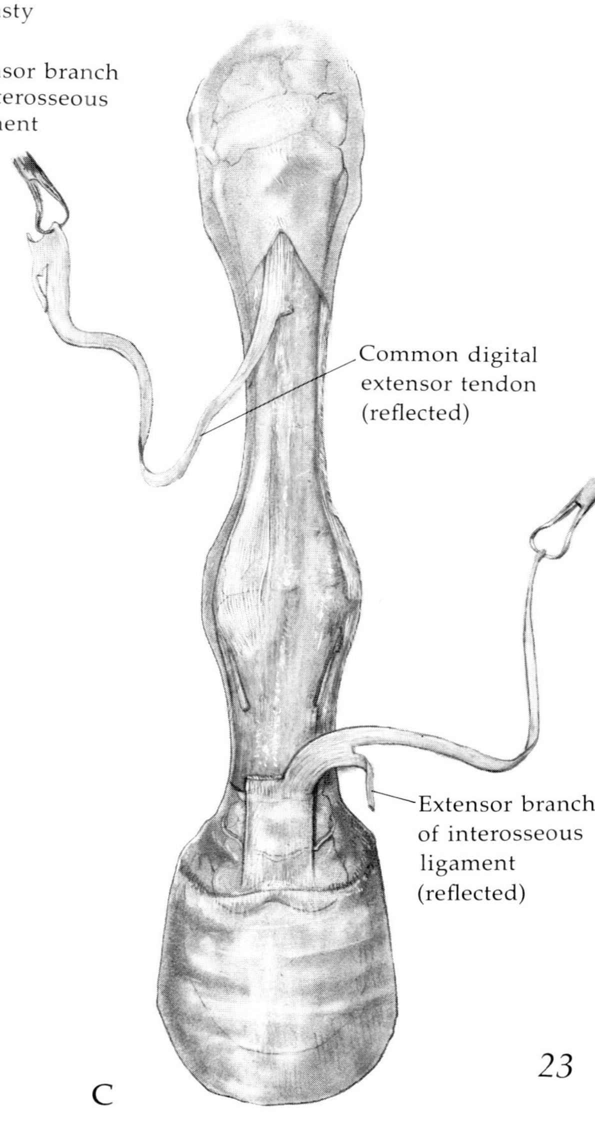

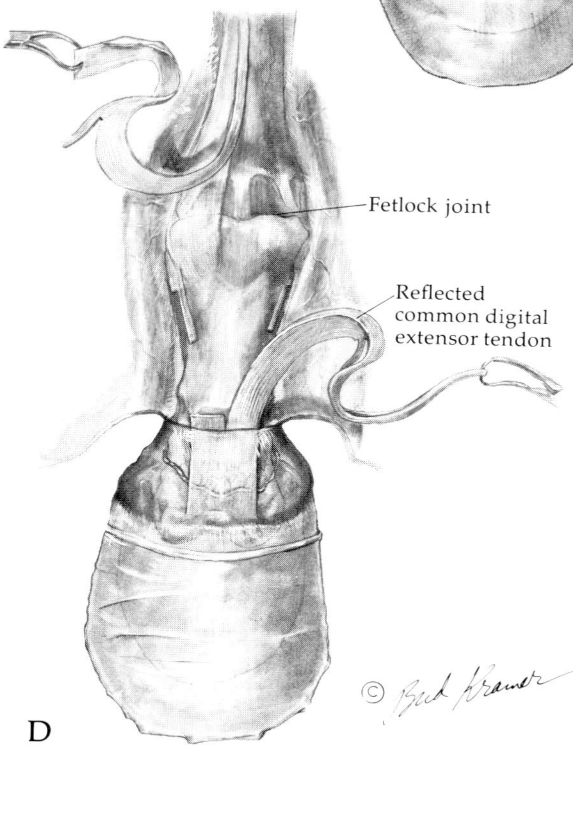

D

C

part three

Approaches to the Proximal Phalanx

LATERAL APPROACH TO PROXIMAL (FIRST) PHALANX

INDICATION

1. Open reduction of the fractures of the proximal phalanx.[1–3]

POSITIONING OF PATIENT

The horse is positioned in right or left lateral recumbency. The configuration of the fracture and the anticipated location of the bone screws will determine whether the affected limb is to the placed up or down.

DESCRIPTION OF PROCEDURE

A. *Topographical View.* A skin incision approximately 7 cm. is made over the lateral aspect of the proximal phalanx. The incision begins 1 cm. distal to the metacarpophalangeal joint to 1 cm. proximal to the proximal interphalangeal joint.

B. *Diagrammatic View of Tendons and Ligaments in Relationship to Bones.* The subcutaneous fascia is incised along the same line as the skin incision, exposing the lateral aspect of the proximal phalanx. The extensor branch of the interosseous (suspensory) ligament passes in a cranial-distal direction over the lateral aspect of the proximal third of the proximal phalanx. It should be visualized and preserved. It can be reflected cranially or caudally to expose the proximal condyle of the proximal phalanx.

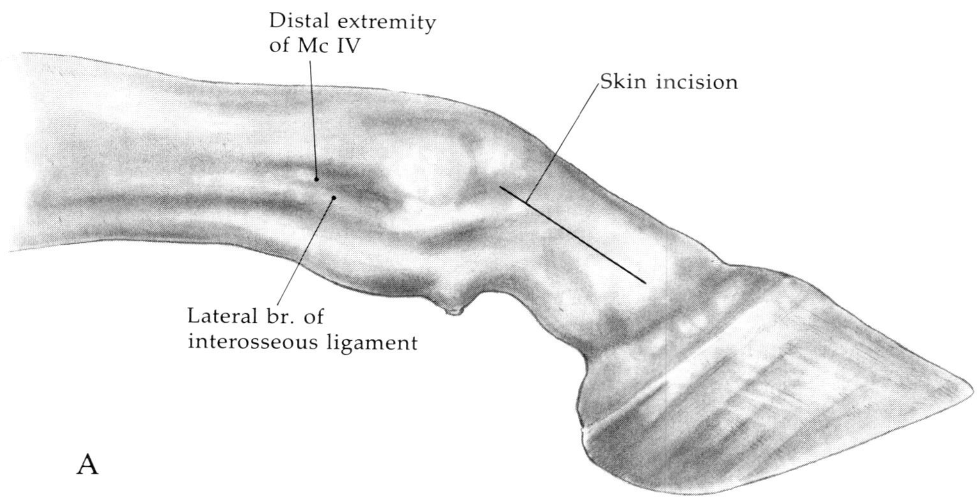
Distal extremity
of Mc IV
Skin incision
Lateral br. of
interosseous ligament

A

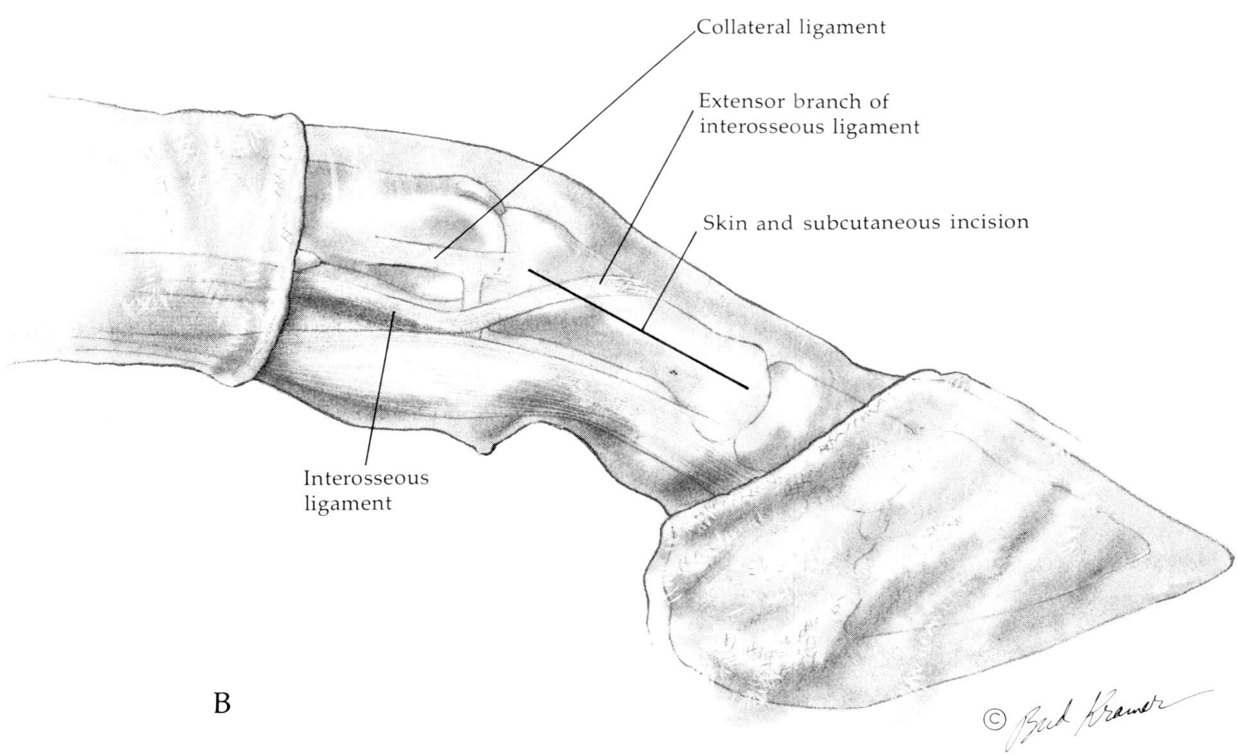
Collateral ligament
Extensor branch of
interosseous ligament
Skin and subcutaneous incision
Interosseous
ligament
© Bud Kramer

B

C. *Surgeon's View.* Care should be taken to avoid severing the artery of the dorsal branch of the proximal phalanx and its branches as they cross over the lateral and cranial aspects of the proximal phalanx.

CLOSURE

An interrupted or continuous suture pattern is used to close the subcutaneous fascia. The skin should be closed with an interrupted suture pattern with the incised edges in firm apposition.

COMMENTS

Fractures of the first phalanx are relatively common in the horse.[1–3] The approach described is applicable to the front or hind limbs, medial or lateral side.

Numerous small stab incisions in the skin, subcutaneous fascia and periosteum at the site of placement of interfragmentary screws may be used instead of the extensive skin incision described, if only one or two interfragmentary screws are being utilized. For repair of the long sagittal fractures, where three or more interfragmentary screws are being inserted, the extensive incision should be utilized, as it gives clear visualization of the extensor branch of the suspensory ligament and the artery of the dorsal branch of the proximal phalanx.

References

1. Bohn, D., and Waibl, H.: Fractures of the First Phalanx in the Horse. Tierztl. Wschr. *90*(1977): 273–175.
2. Dubs, B., and Nemeth, F.: Therapy and Prognosis of First Phalanx Fractures. Schweiz. Arch. Tierheilkd. *117*(1975): 299–309.
3. Fackelman, G. E.: Sagittal Fractures of the First Phalanx (P_1) in the Horse. Vet. Med. Small Anim. Clin. *68*(6):(1973): 622–636.

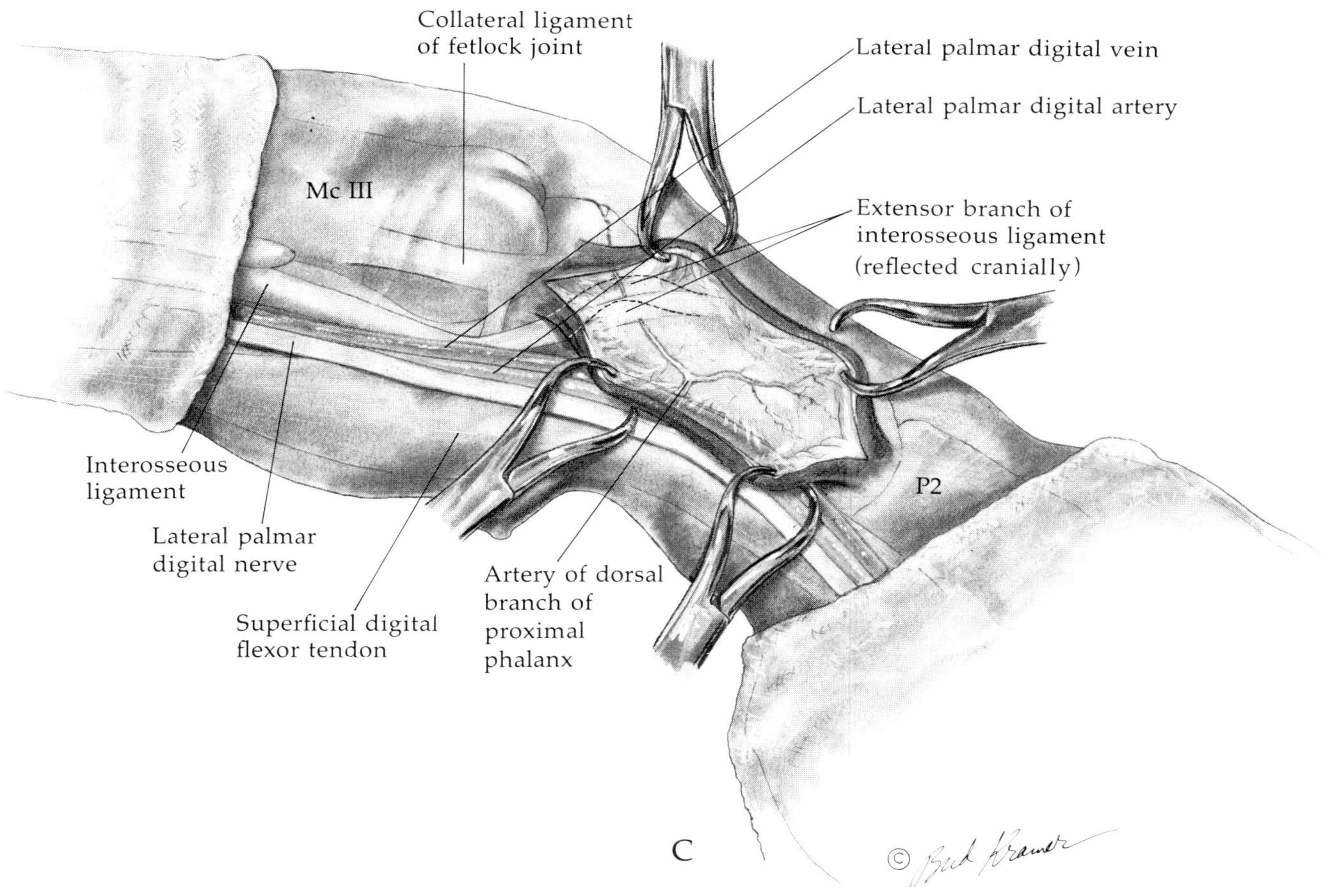
Collateral ligament of fetlock joint
Lateral palmar digital vein
Lateral palmar digital artery
Mc III
Extensor branch of interosseous ligament (reflected cranially)
Interosseous ligament
Lateral palmar digital nerve
Superficial digital flexor tendon
Artery of dorsal branch of proximal phalanx
P2
C
© Bud Kramer

CRANIAL APPROACH TO PROXIMAL PHALANX

INDICATIONS

1. Surgical repair of fractures of the first phalanx.
2. Arthrodesis of the proximal interphalangeal joint.

POSITIONING OF PATIENT

The horse is positioned in right or left lateral recumbency with the affected limb uppermost.

DESCRIPTION OF PROCEDURE

A. *Topographical View.* An I-shaped incision approximately 9 cm. long is made over the cranial surface of the first phalanx. The proximal part of the incision extends across the fetlock joint at the proximal level of the first phalanx. The distal part of the incision is placed across the proximal border of the second phalanx.* The two incisions are connected by a sagittal incision down the cranial aspect of the proximal phalanx.

B. *Surgeon's View.* The skin is reflected medially and laterally from the midline exposing the common digital extensor tendon and the two extensor branches of the interosseous (suspensory) ligaments. A Z-plasty is performed in the common extensor tendon and the two extensor branches of the interosseous ligament. If adequate exposure is obtained after Z-plasty of the common digital extensor tendon, then Z-plasties in the extensor branches of the interosseous ligament may not be necessary.

C. *Surgeon's View.* The tendons are reflected from the cranial surface of the first phalanx. This exposes the underlying bone and fetlock joint capsule.

CLOSURE

The incisions in the tendons are reapposed using a simple interrupted suture pattern with a nonabsorbable suture material. The skin is closed with an interrupted suture pattern with the incised edges in firm apposition.

COMMENTS

The skin on the cranial surface of the proximal phalanx lacks mobility. Placing metal implants on the cranial surface of the first phalanx beneath this nonmobile skin predisposes to postoperative wound dehiscence. Therefore, during surgery, the surgeon must be meticulous in protecting the skin flaps from inadvertent trauma which may further predispose to postoperative wound dehiscence.

For arthrodesis of the proximal interphalangeal joint, the distal part of the I-shaped incision is placed more distally, to just above the coronary band.

To expose the proximal interphalangeal joint for arthrodesis, the joint is opened transversely and placed in flexion.

---

*See Comments.

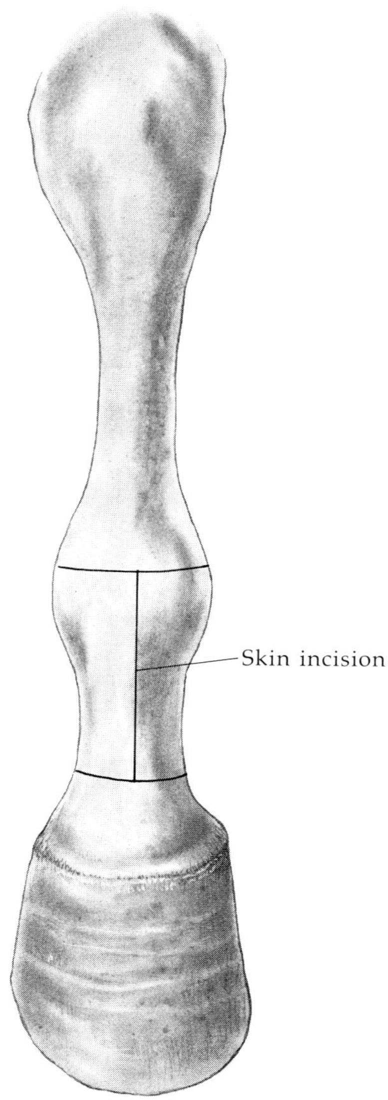
Skin incision

A

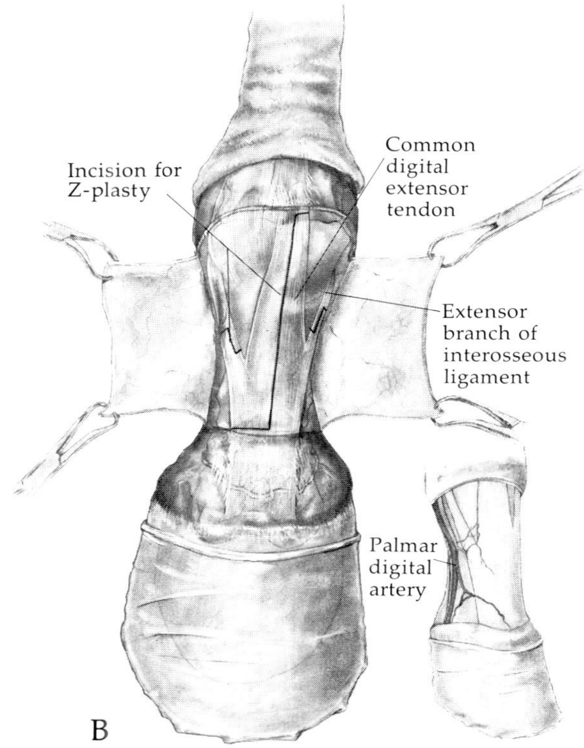
Incision for
Z-plasty
Common
digital
extensor
tendon
Extensor
branch of
interosseous
ligament
Palmar
digital
artery

B

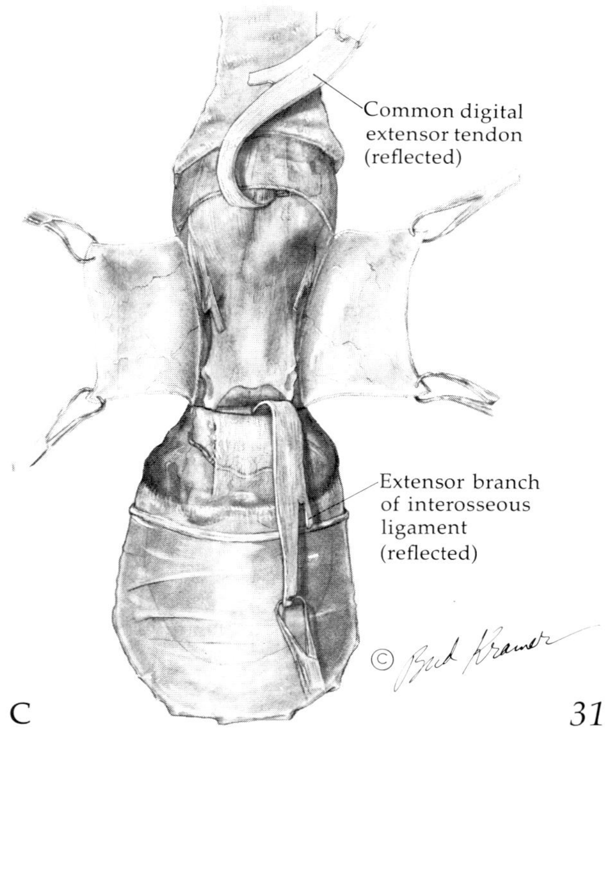
Common digital
extensor tendon
(reflected)
Extensor branch
of interosseous
ligament
(reflected)
© Bud Kramer

C

CRANIAL APPROACH TO FETLOCK JOINT

INDICATIONS

1. Removal of intra-articular chip fractures of the distal aspect of Mc III and proximal aspect of the proximal phalanx (PI).[1, 2, 5]
2. Removal of pedunculated nodular outgrowths of hyperplastic joint capsule (villinodular synovitis).[2, 4]

POSITIONING OF THE PATIENT

The patient is positioned in right or left lateral recumbency with the affected limb down.*

DESCRIPTION OF THE PROCEDURE

A. *Topographical View.* A skin incision approximately 6 cm. long is made 1 cm. medial to the common digital extensor tendon over the fetlock joint. The subcutaneous fascia is incised along the same line as the skin incision.

B. *Surgeon's View.* The incision is continued deep through the joint capsule. The branches of the artery of the dorsal branch of the PI and dorsal branch of palmar metacarpal artery II should be ligated.

C. *Surgeon's View.* The fetlock joint is placed in flexion as the two edges of the incised joint capsule are retracted medially and laterally exposing the articular surfaces of the proximal metacarpophalangeal joint.

CLOSURE

The joint capsule, subcutaneous tissues, and skin should be closed separately. The sutures in the joint capsule should not penetrate the synovial membrane; the synovial membrane of the joint capsule should not be allowed to evert between the opposed edges of the joint capsule, as this reduces the rate and strength of healing.[3] Preplacement of the sutures in the joint capsule will allow a more accurate approximation of the cut edges of the joint capsule and achieve a tight seal (each suture is tied after all sutures have been placed). Interrupted patterns are recommended for closure of the joint capsule. An interrupted or continuous pattern may be used to close the subcutaneous fascia. The skin should be closed with an interrupted pattern, so that the edges are in firm apposition.

---

*See Comments.

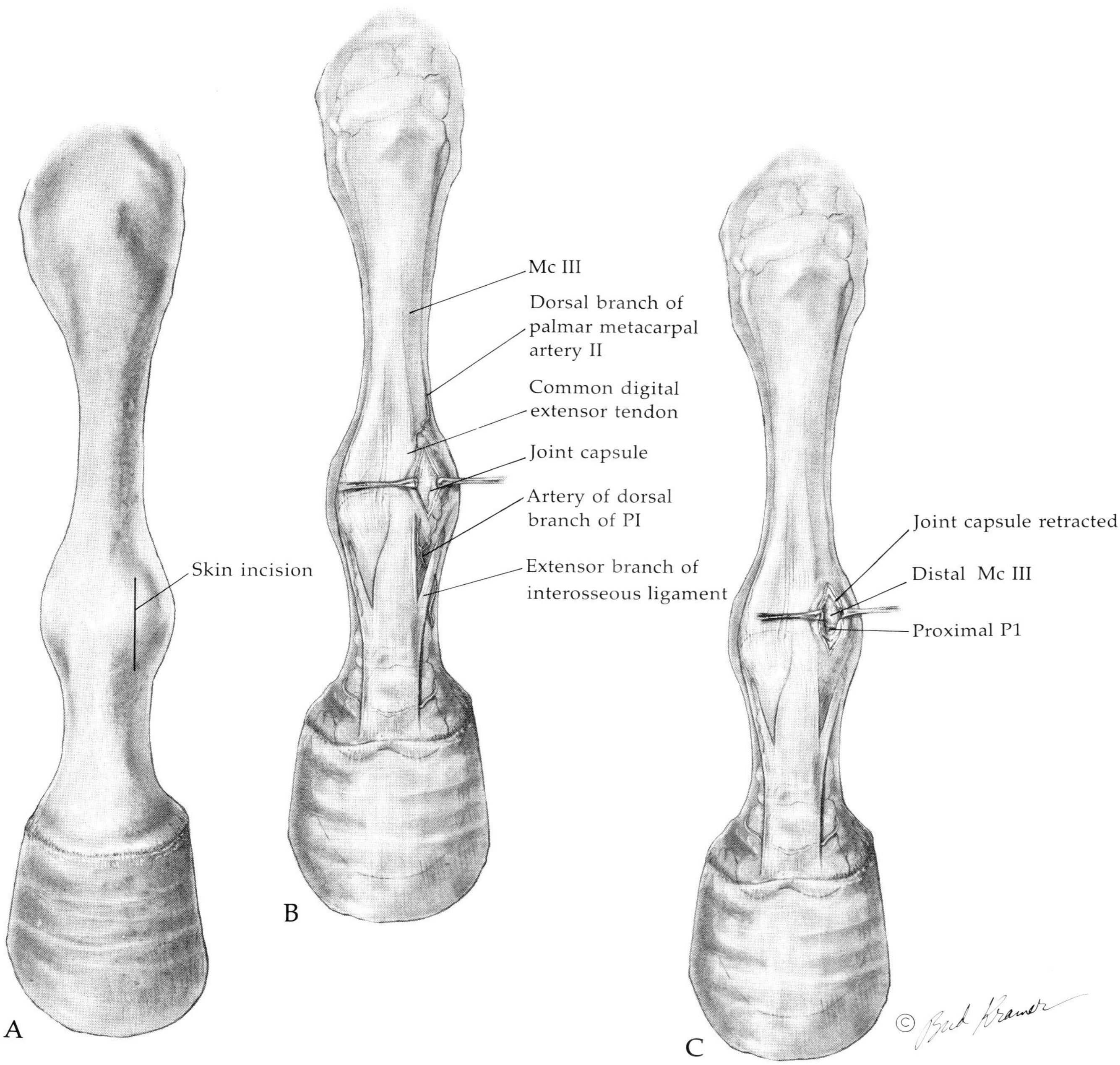
Skin incision
A
Mc III
Dorsal branch of palmar metacarpal artery II
Common digital extensor tendon
Joint capsule
Artery of dorsal branch of PI
Extensor branch of interosseous ligament
B
Joint capsule retracted
Distal Mc III
Proximal P1
C

COMMENTS

Intra-articular chip fractures of the distal aspect of Mc III and the proximal aspect of PI occur more commonly on the medial aspect of the fetlock joint.[1, 2] The approach described is for removal of medial chip fractures. If the chip fracture is lateral, the incision is made 1 cm. lateral to the common digital extensor tendon (the horse is positioned with the affected limb uppermost). Surgical removal of pedunculated nodular growths of the joint capsule can be approached either medial or lateral to the common digital extensor tendon.[4] Occasionally, both incisions may be necessary for complete removal of the mass. A common sequela to surgical repair of intra-articular fractures of the fetlock joint is calcification of the capsule at the periphery of the joint. For this reason conservative, nonsurgical treatment may be indicated.[5]

References

1. Adams, O. R.: Chip Fractures of the First Phalanx in the Metacarpophalangeal (fetlock) Joint. J.A.V.M.A. *148*(4) (1966):360–363.
2. Adams, O. R.: Lameness in Horses. 3rd ed., Philadelphia, Lea and Febiger, 1974, pp. 225–228.
3. International Symposium of Sutures in Wound Repair, London, England, Ethicon, U.S.A. July, 1972.
4. Nickels, F. A., Grant, B. D., and Lincoln, S. D.: Villinodular Synovitis of the Equine Metacarpophalangeal Joint. J.A.V.M.A. 168(11)(1976):1043–1046.
5. Raker, C. W.: Calcification of the Equine Metacarpophalangeal Joint Following Removal of Chip Fractures. Arch. Am. Coll. Vet. Surg. (Spring 1975):66–68.

part four

Approaches to the Proximal Sesamoid Bones

LATERAL (CHURCHILL) APPROACH TO PROXIMAL SESAMOID BONE

INDICATIONS

1. Surgical excision of apical sesamoid fractures.[1, 2, 4, 8, 10]
2. Surgical excision of basilar sesamoid fractures.[6, 9]
3. Open reduction and fixation of sesamoid fractures (in combination with basilar approach to the proximal sesamoid).[3, 7]

POSITIONING OF PATIENT

The horse is placed in either right or left lateral recumbency, depending on whether the medial or lateral sesamoid is to be approached. The limb is maintained in an extended position (dorsiflexion) while entering the joint. By maintaining the limb in extension while making the incision, the anatomical structures (flexor tendons and interosseous [suspensory] ligament) are more obvious. This makes it easier for the surgeon to place his incision correctly. Once the joint has been entered, placing the limb in flexion will allow good exposure of the articular surface of the proximal sesamoid bone.

DESCRIPTION OF PROCEDURE

A. *Topographical View.* An incision approximately 5 cm. long is made over the lateral cul-de-sac of the fetlock joint caudal to the caudal border of Mc III and cranial to the cranial border of the interosseous ligament. The incision begins 1 cm. distal to the distal extremity of the fourth metacarpus (Mc IV) and extends to the proximal border of the lateral collateral sesamoidean ligament. The subcutaneous fascia is incised on the same line as the skin incision.

B. *Diagrammatic View of Tendons and Ligaments in Relation to Bones.* An incision approximately 3.5 cm. long is made through the joint capsule, extending from approximately 2 cm. distal to the distal extremity of Mc IV to approximately 0.5 cm. proximal to the proximal border of the lateral collateral sesamoidean ligament.

C. *Surgeon's View.* The incision through the joint capsule should not normally extend through the lateral collateral sesamoidean ligament.* The fetlock joint is placed in flexion as the two edges of the joint capsule are retracted cranially and caudally. This exposes the caudal articular surface of the third metacarpus and the articular surface of the proximal sesamoid bone.

---

*See Comments.

LATERAL (CHURCHILL) APPROACH TO PROXIMAL SESAMOID BONE

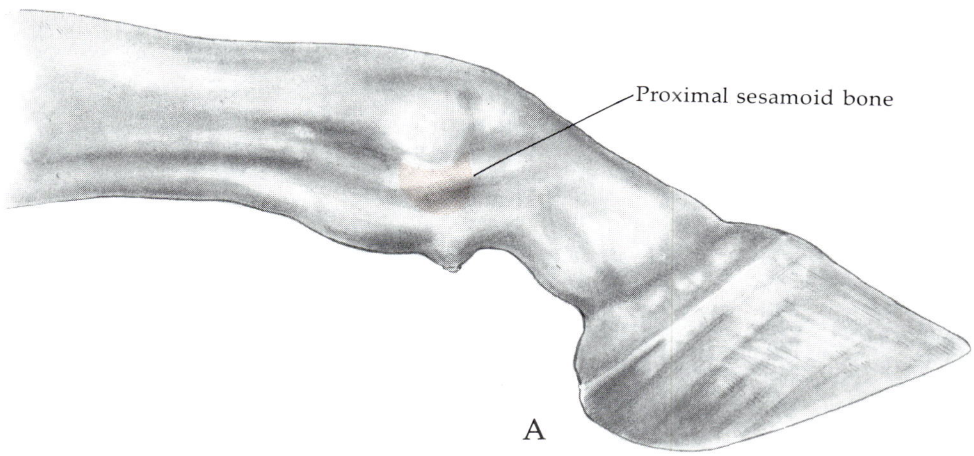

A

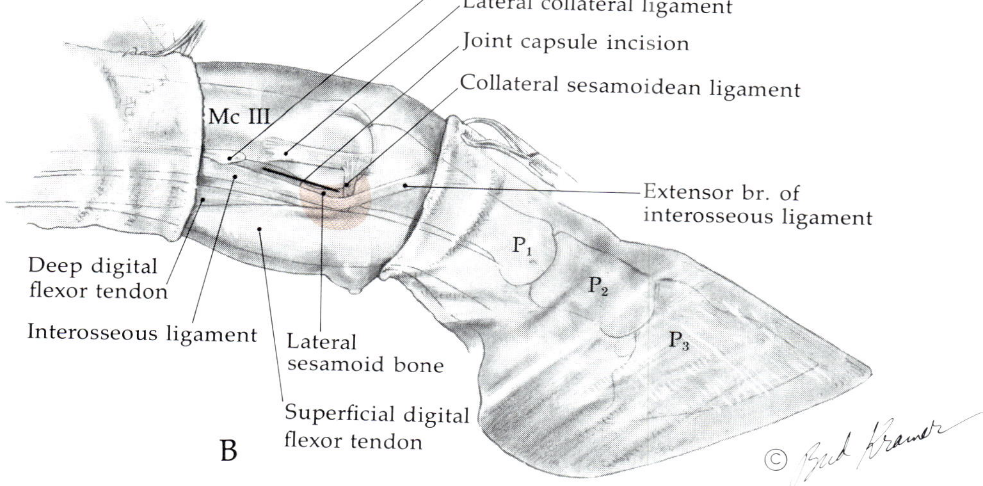

B

LATERAL (CHURCHILL) APPROACH TO PROXIMAL SESAMOID BONE

D. Surgeon's View. Care should be taken when extending the incision in the joint capsule proximally because of its relationship to the arteries of the palmar arch. If the incision is extended too far proximally, extensive hemorrhage will occur. The dorsal and palmar branches of the palmar metacarpal artery extend through the proximal aspect of the joint capsule. The transected branches of these arteries to the joint capsule should be carefully ligated.

CLOSURE

The joint capsule, subcutaneous fascia, and skin should be closed separately. The sutures in the joint capsule should not penetrate the synovial membrane; the synovial membrane of the joint capsule should not be allowed to evert between the opposed edges of the fibrous joint capsule, as this reduces the rate and strength of healing.[5] Preplacement of all the sutures in the joint capsule will allow a more accurate approximation of the cut edges of the joint capsule and achieve a tight seal (each individual suture is tied after all sutures have been placed). Interrupted suture patterns are recommended for closure of the joint capsule. An interrupted or continuous suture pattern should be used to close the subcutaneous fascia.

The skin should be closed with an interrupted suture pattern with the incised edges in firm apposition.

COMMENTS

Surgical excision of apical fractures of the proximal sesamoid bone was one of the first procedures developed in joint surgery in the horse.[2] The diagnosis, treatment, and prognosis of fractures of the proximal sesamoids have been described.[1–4, 8–10] The approaches to the lateral and medial sesamoid are essentially the same.

When surgical excision of basilar fractures of the proximal sesamoid is indicated, the incision can be extended distally through the lateral collateral sesamoidean ligament to provide more exposure to the articular surface of the sesamoid. Alternatively, the caudal approach to the proximal sesamoid bone can be used. For open reduction of sesamoid fractures a combination of the lateral and the basilar approaches should be used. This enables the articular surface of the proximal sesamoid bone to be visualized during reduction and fixation.

References

1. Adams, O. R.: Lameness in Horses. 3rd ed., Philadelphia, Lea and Febiger, 1974, pp. 219–225.
2. Churchill, E. A.: Surgical Removal of Fractured Fragments of the Proximal Sesamoid Bone. J.A.V.M.A.*128*(1956): 581–582.
3. Fackelman, G. E.: Compression Screw Fixation of Proximal Sesamoid Fractures. J. Equine Med. Surg. 2:(1978): 32–39.
4. Hernze, C. D.: Equine Orthopedic Surgery. Mod. Vet. Pract. (Red Book) (October 15, 1966), pp. 63–84.
5. International Symposium of Sutures in Wound Repair. London, England, Ethicon, U.S.A. July, 1972.
6. Larson, L. H., Dixon, R. T., and Heron, J.: Surgical Treatment of Fractures of the Proximal Sesamoid Bones in the Horse. Aust. Vet. J. *40*(1964): 203–213.
7. McKibbin, L. S., and Armstrong, K. N.: Bone Screws As A Method For Immobilizing Sesamoid Fragments. Proceedings American Association of Equine Practitioners, (1970): 203–206.
8. Sevelius, F., and Tufuesson, G.: Treatment for Fractures of the Sesamoid Bones in Horses. J.A.V.M.A. *142*(1963): 981–988.
9. Wheat, J. D., and Rhode, E. A.: The Surgical Treatment of Fractures of the Proximal Sesamoid Bones in the Horse. J.A.V.M.A. *132*(1958): 378–382.
10. Wirstad, H. F.: Fractures of the Proximal Phalangeal Sesamoid Bones. Vet. Rec. *75*(1963): 509–513.

LATERAL (CHURCHILL) APPROACH TO PROXIMAL SESAMOID BONE

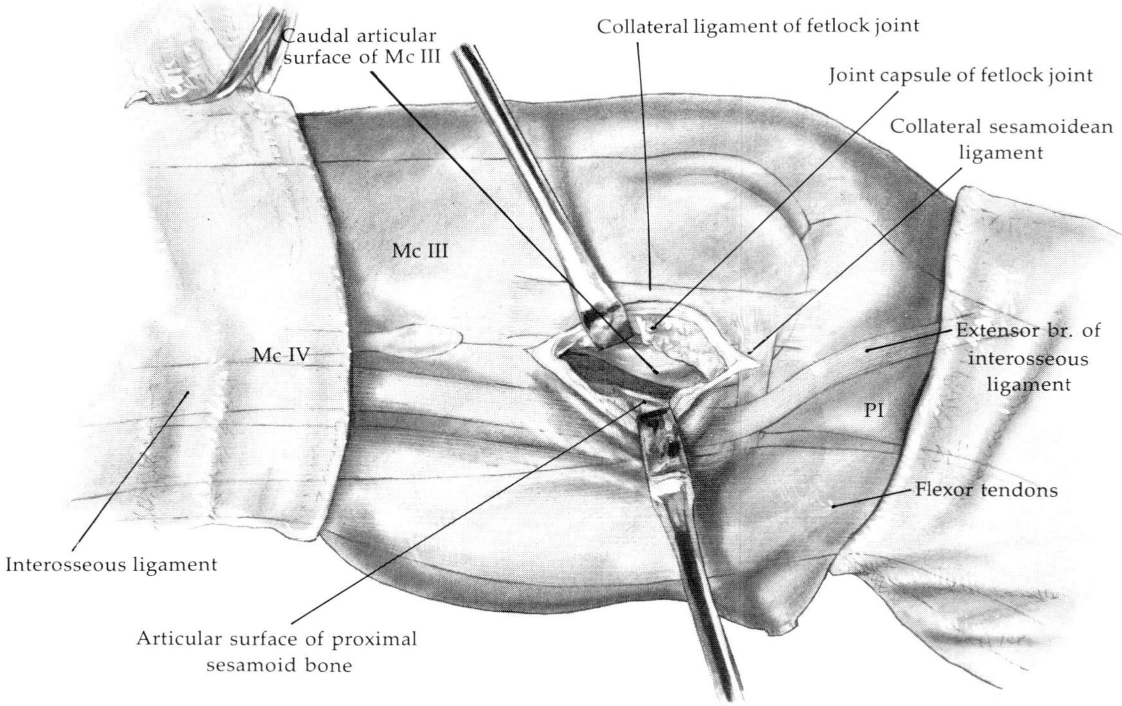

C

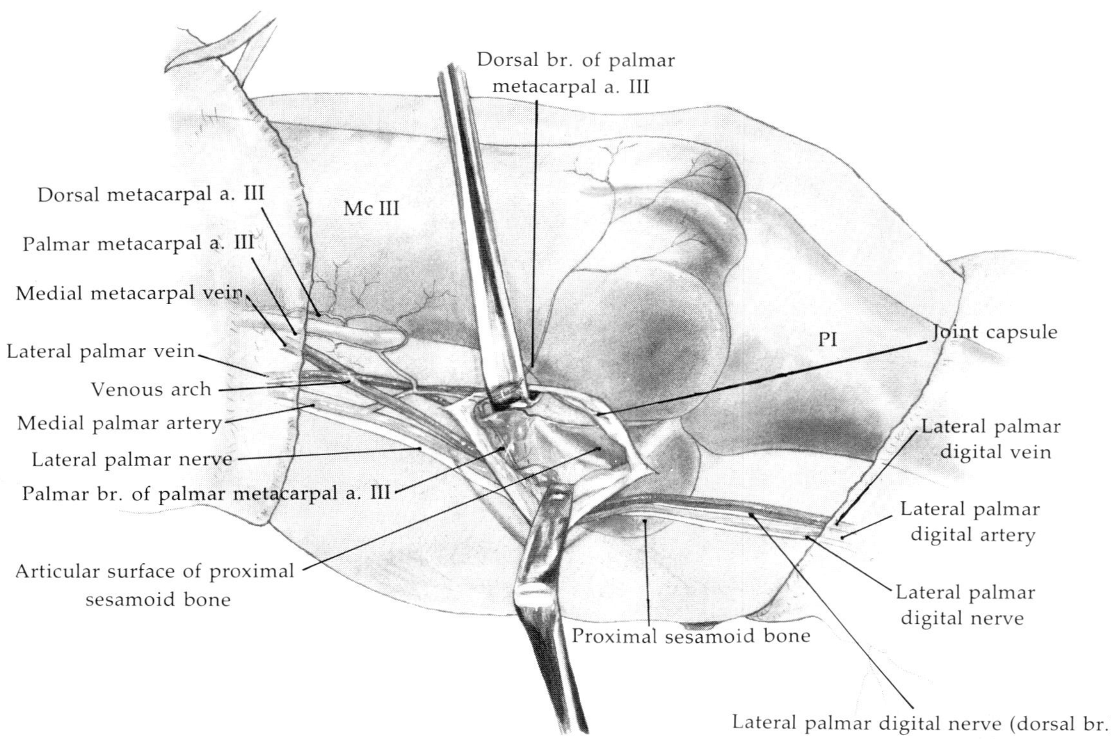

D

BASILAR APPROACH TO PROXIMAL SESAMOID BONE

INDICATIONS

1. Open reduction of sesamoid fractures.[3, 4]
2. Surgical excision of basilar sesamoid fractures.[1, 2, 5]

POSITIONING OF PATIENT

The horse is placed in either right or left lateral recumbency depending on whether the medial or lateral sesamoid is to be approached. The limb is maintained in an extended position (dorsiflexion) while the incision is made. By maintaining the limb in extension, the anatomical structures (flexor tendons, interosseous [suspensory] ligament, and palmar digital artery, vein, and nerve) are more obvious. This makes it easier for the surgeon to place his incision correctly.

DESCRIPTION OF PROCEDURE

A. Topographical View. The surgeon's thumb is used to retract the lateral palmar digital artery, vein, and nerve cranially, so that the skin incision can be made without excising these structures. A skin incision of approximately 6 cm. is made over the base of the sesamoid, extending from the middle of the lateral aspect of the sesamoid to just beyond the distal border of the proximal branch of the digital annular ligament. The subcutaneous fascia is incised on the same line as the skin incision.

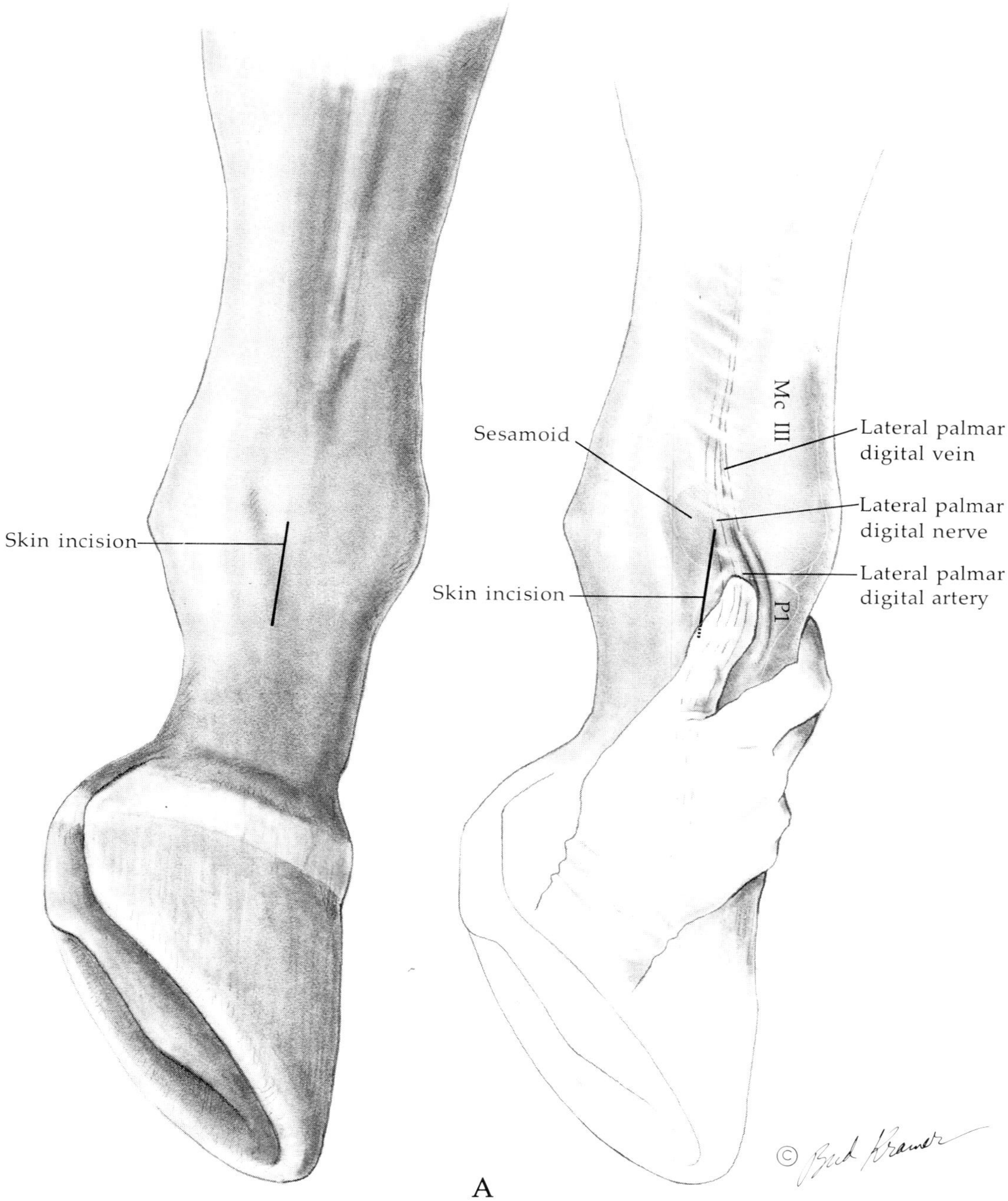
Skin incision
Sesamoid
Mc III
Lateral palmar digital vein
Lateral palmar digital nerve
Lateral palmar digital artery
Skin incision
P1
© Bud Kramer

A

B. *Diagrammatic View of Tendons and Ligaments in Relationship to Bones.* Once the skin and subcutaneous fascia are incised and retracted, the distal edge of the volar annular ligament and the cranial edge of the tendon sheath of the deep flexor tendon are exposed. These structures form a triangular space into which deeper dissection is continued to the base of the sesamoid bone (the triangle is formed by the distal edge of the volar annular ligament proximally, the proximal edge of the proximal branch of the digital annular ligament distally, and the cranial edge of the tendon sheath of the deep flexor tendon caudally).

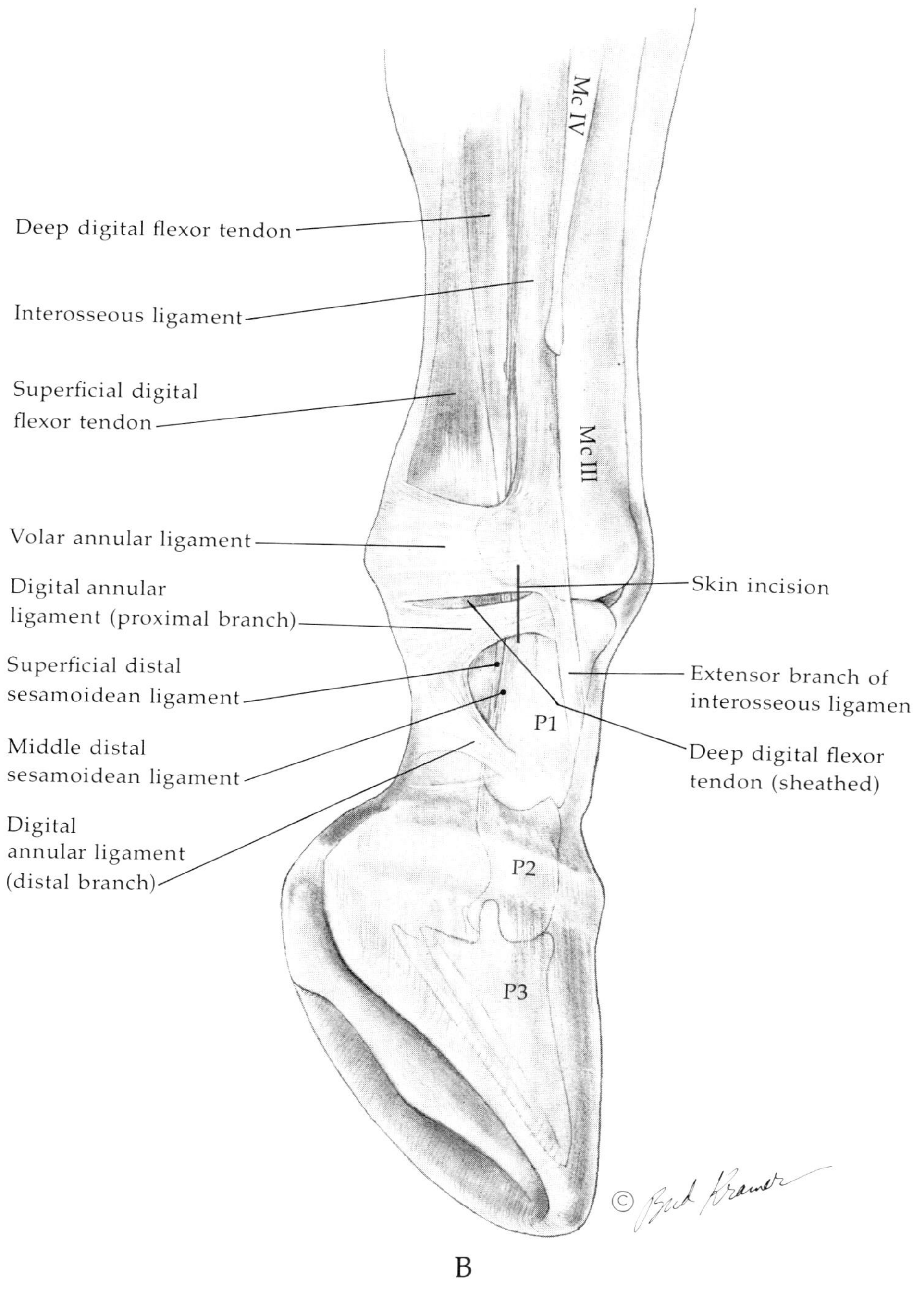
Mc IV
Deep digital flexor tendon
Interosseous ligament
Superficial digital flexor tendon
Mc III
Volar annular ligament
Skin incision
Digital annular ligament (proximal branch)
Superficial distal sesamoidean ligament
Extensor branch of interosseous ligament
P1
Deep digital flexor tendon (sheathed)
Middle distal sesamoidean ligament
Digital annular ligament (distal branch)
P2
P3
© Bud Kramer

B

C. *Surgeon's View.* Care should be taken to avoid incising the lateral palmar digital artery, vein, and nerve which pass cranially to the incision over the caudal-lateral aspect of the distal Mc III, and proximal PI, and the lateral aspect of the proximal sesamoid (sesamoid screened in red).

D. *Surgeon's View.* To expose the attachments of the superficial and middle distal sesamoidean ligaments a deep incision is made which completely excises the proximal branch of the digital annular ligament, and extends proximally through the distal border of the volar annular ligament for approximately 1 cm. to the level of the base of the proximal sesamoid. Care should be taken to avoid incising the tendon sheath of the flexor tendons which lies in close apposition to the superficial distal sesamoidean ligament.

E. The base of the proximal sesamoid is exposed by separating the superficial distal sesamoidean and middle distal sesamoidean ligaments. The superficial distal sesamoidean ligament is retracted caudally, and the middle distal sesamoidean ligament is retracted cranially.

CLOSURE

The proximal branch of the digital annular ligament is reapposed using an interrupted suture pattern. An interrupted or continuous suture pattern should be used to close the subcutaneous fascia. The skin should be closed with an interrupted suture pattern with the incised edges in firm apposition.

COMMENTS

When open reduction of sesamoid fractures is to be performed, this approach is used in combination with the lateral approach to the proximal sesamoid bone. This enables the articular surface of the proximal sesamoid bone to be visualized during reduction and fixation.

Some surgeons may prefer a stab incision extending through the triangle formed by the distal edge of the volar annular ligament proximally, the proximal edge of the proximal branch of the digital annular ligament distally, and the cranial edge of the tendon sheath of the flexor tendons caudally. However, that method prevents visualization of important anatomical structures.

References

1. Adams, O. R.: Lameness in Horses. 3rd ed., Philadelphia, Lea and Febiger, 1974, pp. 219–225.
2. Larson, L. H., Dixon, R. T., and Heron, J.: Surgical Treatment of Fractures of the Proximal Sesamoid Bones in the Horse. Aust. Vet. J. *40* (1964): 203–213.
3. Fackelman, G. E.: Compression Screw Fixation of Proximal Sesamoid Fractures. J. Equine Med. Surg. *2* (1978): 32–39.
4. McKibbin, L. S., and Armstrong, K. N.: Bone Screws as a Method for Immobilizing Sesamoid Fragments. Proceedings, 16th Annual Convention, American Association of Equine Practitioners. (1970):203–206.
5. Wheat, J. D., and Rhode, E. A.: The Surgical Treatment of Fractures of the Proximal Sesamoid Bones in the Horse. J.A.V.M.A. *132* (1958): 378–382.

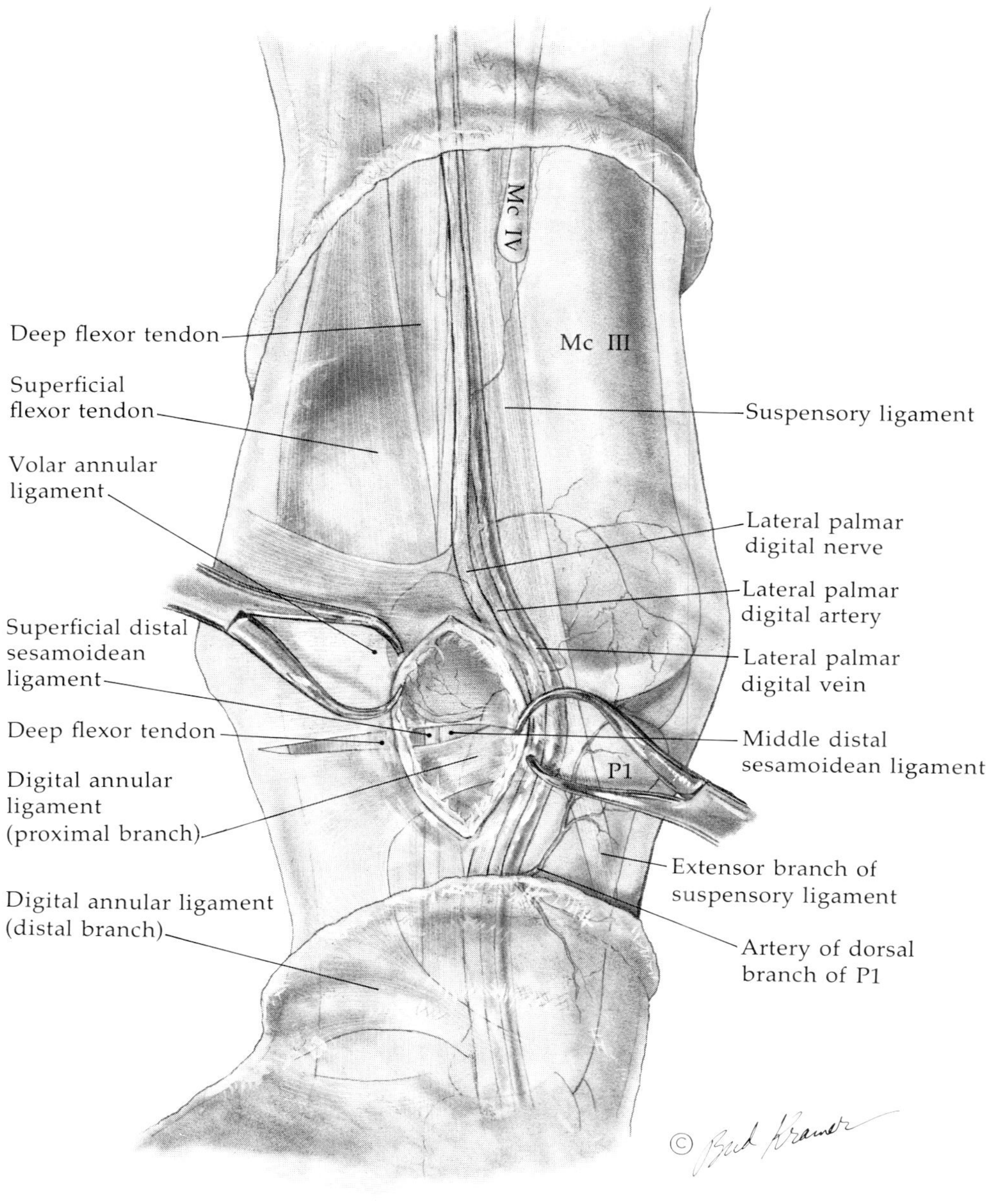
Mc IV
Mc III
Deep flexor tendon
Superficial flexor tendon
Suspensory ligament
Volar annular ligament
Lateral palmar digital nerve
Lateral palmar digital artery
Superficial distal sesamoidean ligament
Lateral palmar digital vein
Deep flexor tendon
Middle distal sesamoidean ligament
P1
Digital annular ligament (proximal branch)
Extensor branch of suspensory ligament
Digital annular ligament (distal branch)
Artery of dorsal branch of P1

C

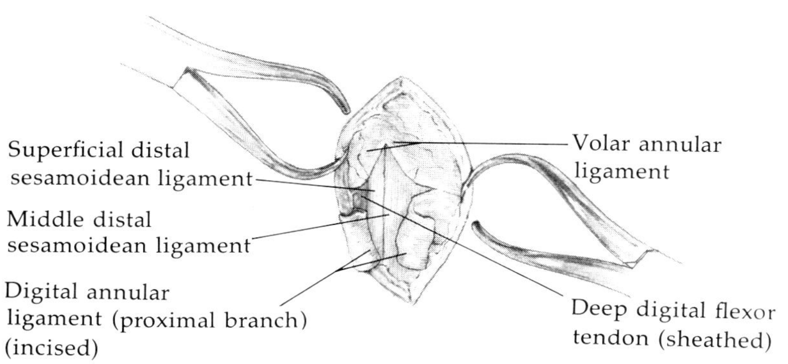
Superficial distal sesamoidean ligament
Volar annular ligament
Middle distal sesamoidean ligament
Digital annular ligament (proximal branch) (incised)
Deep digital flexor tendon (sheathed)

D

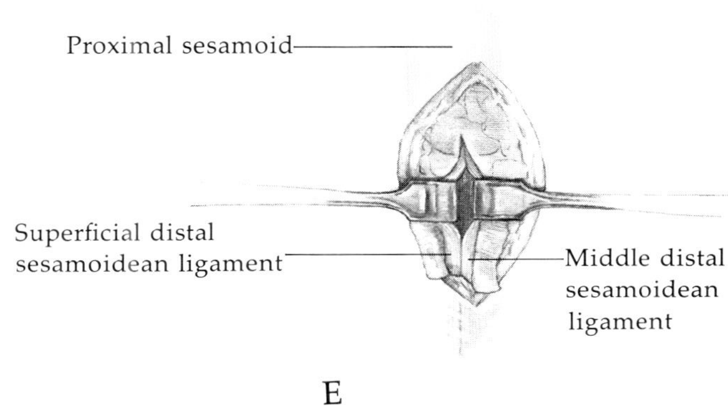
Proximal sesamoid
Superficial distal sesamoidean ligament
Middle distal sesamoidean ligament

E

CAUDAL APPROACH TO THE PROXIMAL SESAMOID BONE

INDICATION

1. Surgical excision of basilar sesamoid fractures.[1–3]

POSITIONING OF PATIENT

The horse is placed in either right or left lateral recumbency, with the affected sesamoid bone uppermost. The limb is maintained in an extended position (dorsiflexion) while the incision is made. When the limb is maintained in extension, the anatomical structures (flexor tendons and interosseous ligament) are more obvious, thus making it easier for the surgeon to place his incision correctly.

DESCRIPTION OF PROCEDURE

A. *Topographical View.* A skin incision approximately 6 cm. is made caudal to the caudal-lateral aspect of the proximal sesamoid bone (proximal sesamoid bones screened in red) extending from above the proximal border to below the distal border of the volar annular ligament. The incision lies caudal to the caudal-lateral border of the deep flexor tendon.

B. *Diagrammatic View of Tendons and Ligaments in Relationship to Bones.* The subcutaneous fascia is incised along the same line as the skin incision, exposing the volar annular ligament.

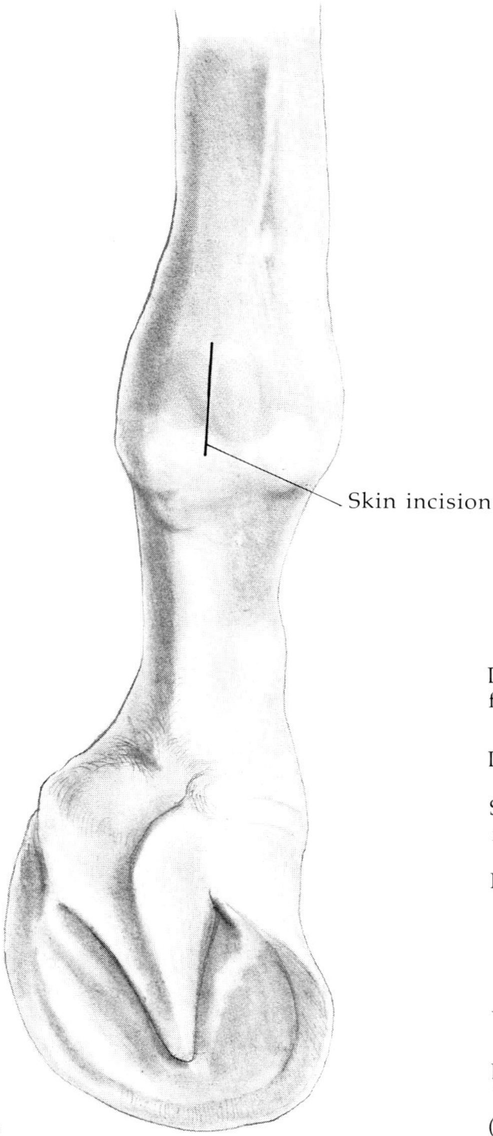
Skin incision

A

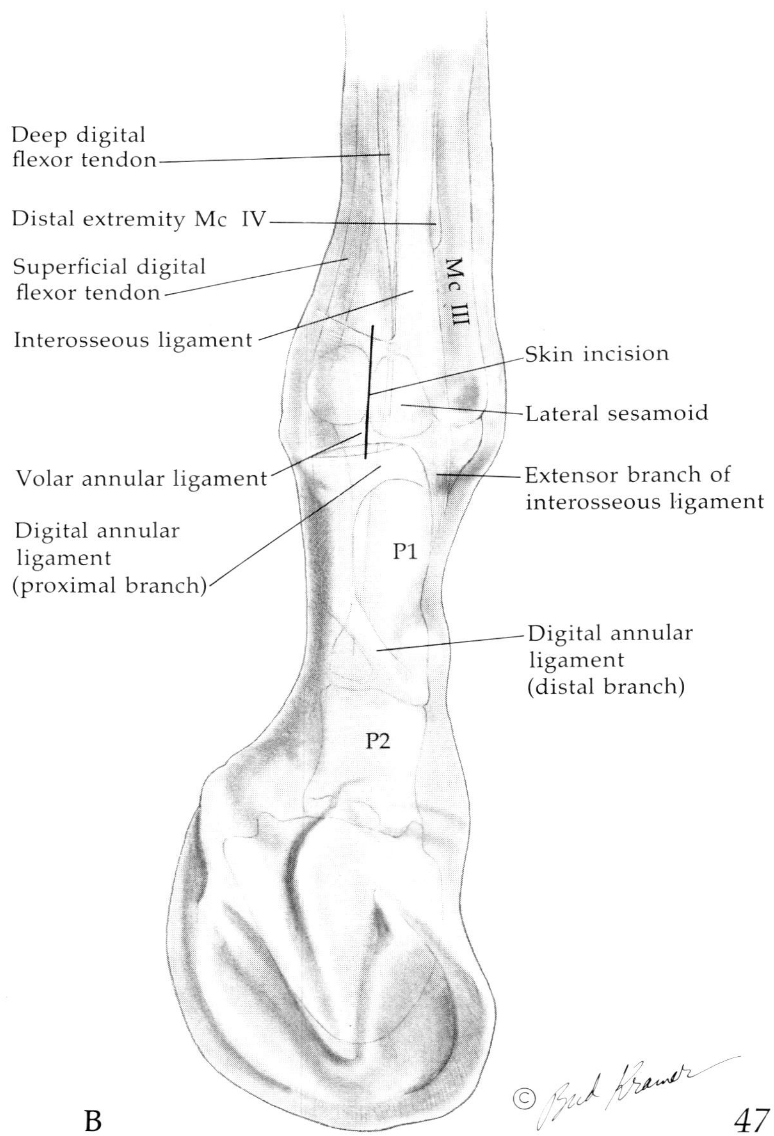
Deep digital flexor tendon
Distal extremity Mc IV
Superficial digital flexor tendon
Interosseous ligament
Volar annular ligament
Digital annular ligament (proximal branch)
Mc III
Skin incision
Lateral sesamoid
Extensor branch of interosseous ligament
P1
Digital annular ligament (distal branch)
P2

B

C. *Surgeon's View.* When making the incision through the skin and subcutaneous fascia, care should be taken to avoid the lateral palmar digital nerve, artery, and vein, which lie lateral to the caudal-lateral border of the proximal sesamoid.

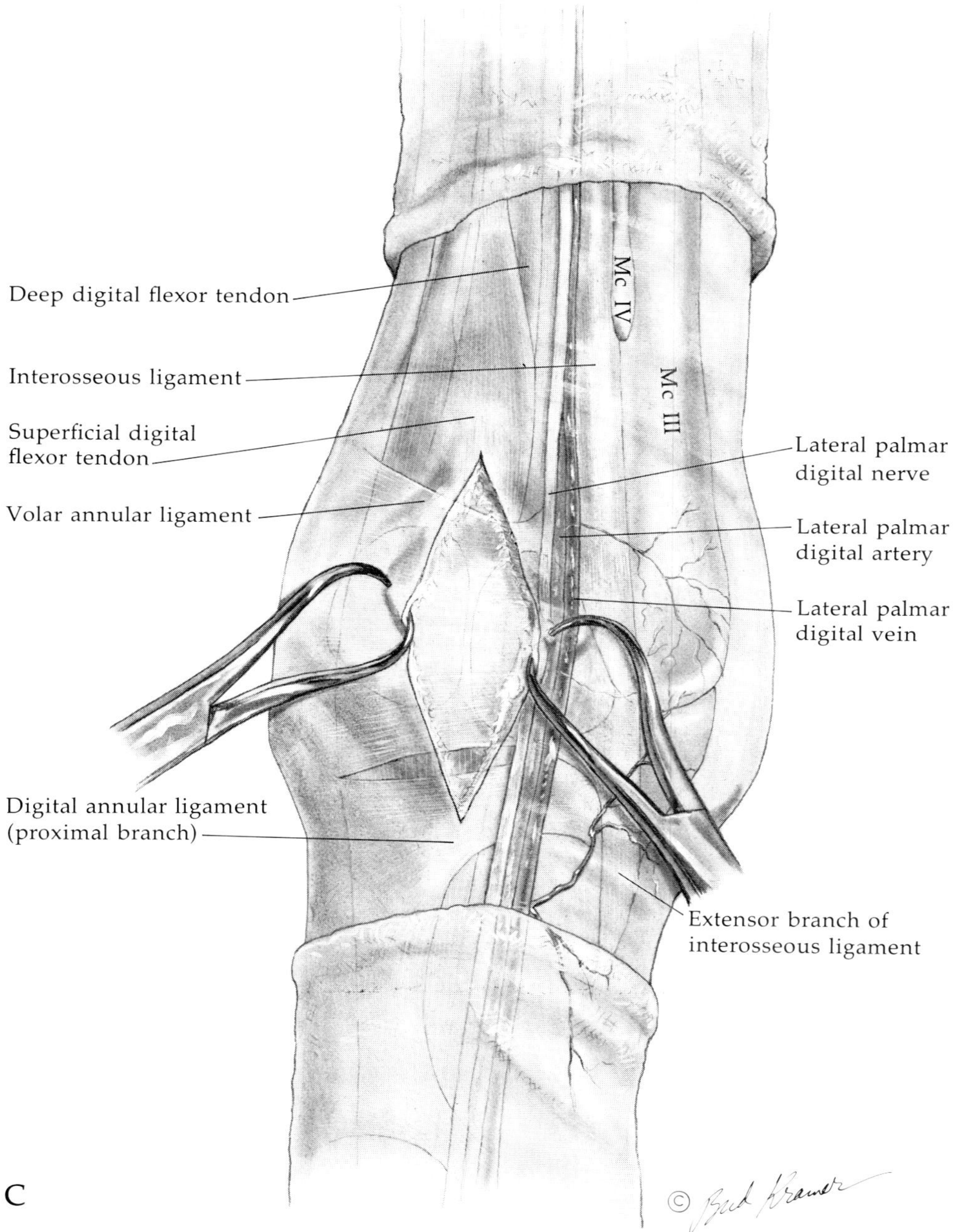
Deep digital flexor tendon
Interosseous ligament
Superficial digital flexor tendon
Volar annular ligament
Digital annular ligament (proximal branch)
Mc IV
Mc III
Lateral palmar digital nerve
Lateral palmar digital artery
Lateral palmar digital vein
Extensor branch of interosseous ligament
© Bud Kramer

C

D. *Surgeon's View.* The volar annular ligament is incised from its proximal to distal border, exposing the deep and superficial flexor tendons. The deep and superficial flexor tendons are retracted caudomedially, exposing the intersesamoidean ligament. This ligament extends from the axial border of the lateral sesamoid to the axial border of the medial sesamoid. This also exposes the attachments of the distal sesamoidean ligaments arising from the base of the proximal sesamoid bone.

CLOSURE

The volar annular ligament is closed using an interrupted suture pattern. The subcutaneous fascia is closed with an interrupted or continuous suture pattern. The skin should be closed with an interrupted suture pattern so that the incised edges are in firm apposition.

COMMENTS

To excise basilar fractures of the proximal sesamoid, it is necessary to sever the attachments of the distal sesamoidean ligaments from the base of the sesamoid.[1–3]

References

1. Adams, O. R.: Lameness in Horses. 3rd ed., Philadelphia, Lea and Febiger, 1974, pp. 219–225.
2. Larson, L. H., Dixon, R. T., and Heron, J.: Surgical Treatment of Fractures of the Proximal Sesamoid Bones in the Horse. Aust. Vet. J. *40* (1964): 203–213.
3. Wheat, J. D., and Rhode, E. A.: The Surgical Treatment of Fractures of the Proximal Sesamoid Bones in the Horse. J.A.V.M.A. *132* (1958): 378–382.

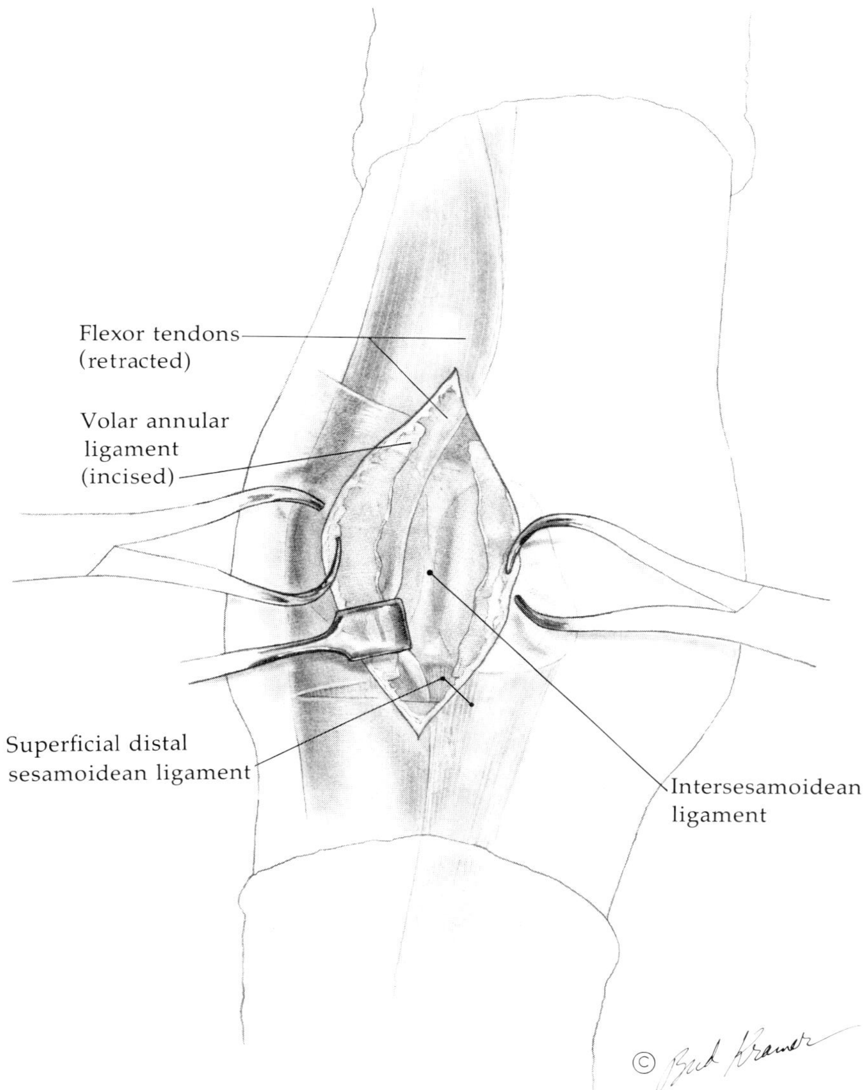
Flexor tendons
(retracted)
Volar annular
ligament
(incised)
Superficial distal
sesamoidean ligament
Intersesamoidean
ligament
© Bud Kramer

D

part five

Approaches to the Second and Third Metacarpal Bones

LATERAL APPROACH TO DISTAL CONDYLE OF Mc III (THIRD METACARPUS)

INDICATION

1. Open reduction of lateral distal condylar fractures of the third metacarpus.[1,2,4]

POSITIONING OF PATIENT

The horse is positioned in left or right lateral recumbency with the affected side of the limb uppermost.

DESCRIPTION OF PROCEDURE

A. *Topographical View.* A skin incision approximately 8 cm. long is made over the distal-lateral aspect of the Mc III. The incision should begin approximately 1 cm. proximal to the proximal end of the lateral collateral ligament to approximately 1 cm. proximal to the metacarpophalangeal joint.

B. *Diagrammatic View of Ligaments and Tendons in Relationship to Bones.* The subcutaneous fascia is incised down to the lateral collateral ligament of the fetlock joint along the same line as the skin incision.

LATERAL APPROACH TO DISTAL CONDYLE OF Mc III (THIRD METACARPUS)

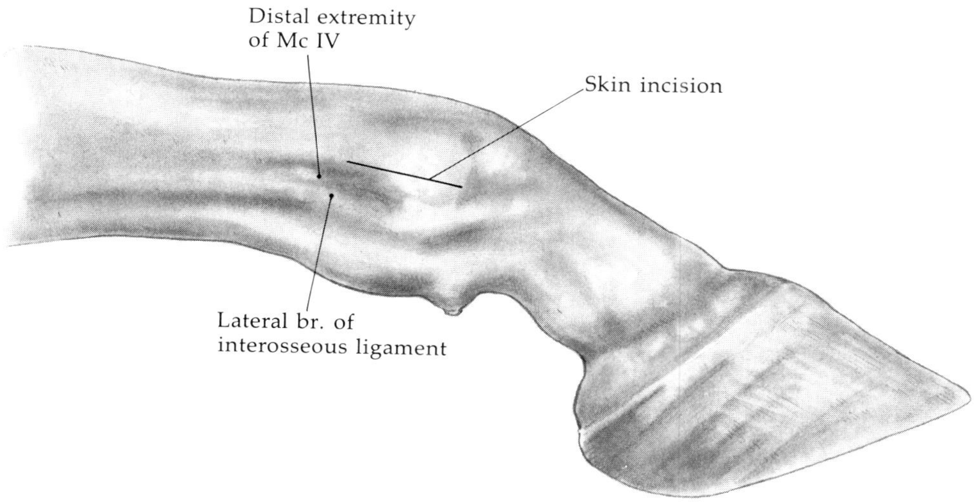

A

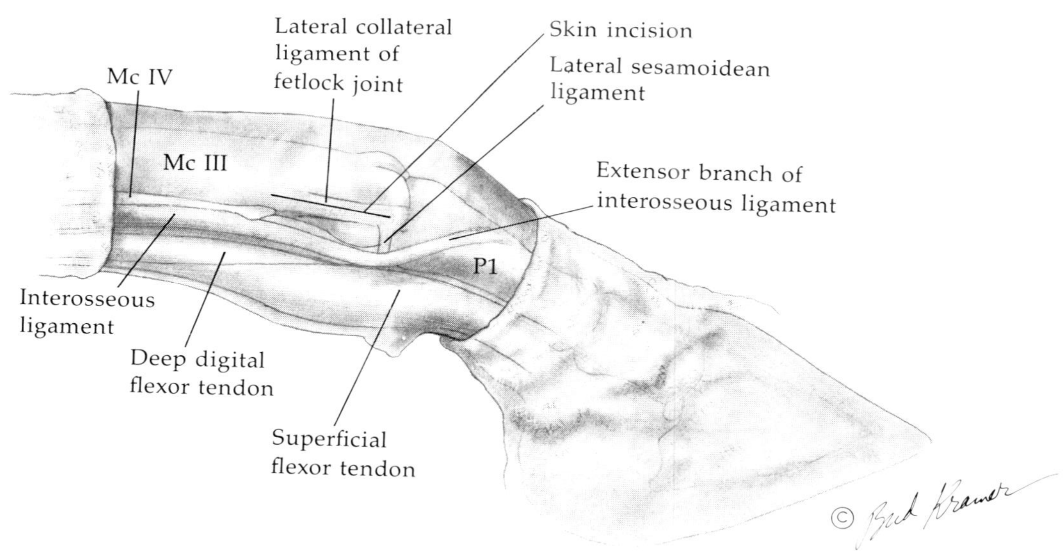

B

C. Surgeon's View. Once the lateral collateral ligament of the fetlock joint is exposed, small stab incisions are made through the ligament down to the bone to place implants for reduction of condylar fractures. The dorsal branch of the palmar metatarsal artery crosses the junction of the proximal and middle third of the collateral ligament. It may be ligated if necessary.

CLOSURE

An interrupted or continuous suture pattern should be used to close the subcutaneous fascia. The skin should be closed with an interrupted suture pattern so that the incised edges are in firm apposition.

COMMENTS

The approach described is applicable to the front or hind limbs, medial or lateral side. Distal condylar fractures usually involve the lateral distal condyle of the third metacarpus.[3] It is seen most commonly in the thoroughbred racehorse.[1-4] The fractures are often repaired with screws, using the lag screw principle with interfragmentary fixation. Numerous small stab incisions through the skin and subcutaneous fascia in the line of the approach described above can be used for the placement of the screws. The advantage of the more extensive incision is clear visualization of the collateral ligament. In addition, visualization and alignment of the proximal end of the fracture will help ensure its alignment at the joint surface. Removal of small fragments of bone that sometimes occur at the proximal end of the fracture is possible with a more liberal skin incision. These fractures often spiral cranially or caudally, and this approach may give the surgeon a better appreciation of the configuration of the fracture. Stab incisions through the collateral ligament are usually necessary for placement of interfragmentary screws to ensure accurate anatomical reduction of the condylar fracture at the articular surface.

References

1. Adams, O. R.: Lameness in Horses. 3rd ed., Philadelphia, Lea and Febiger, 1974, pp. 215–217.
2. Alexander, J. T., and Rooney, J. R.: The Biomechanics, Surgery and Prognosis of Equine Fractures. *In* Proceedings 18th Annual Meeting, American Association Equine Practitioners, 1972. (1973): 219–235.
3. Rooney, J. R.: Distal Condylar Fractures of the Cannon Bone in the Horse. Mod. Vet. Pract. *52* (2) (1974): 113.
4. Meagher, D. M.: Lateral Condylar Fractures of the Metacarpus and Metatarsus in Horses. *In* Proceedings 22nd Annual Meeting, American Association Equine Practitioners, 1976. (1977): 147–154.

LATERAL APPROACH TO DISTAL CONDYLE OF Mc III (THIRD METACARPUS)

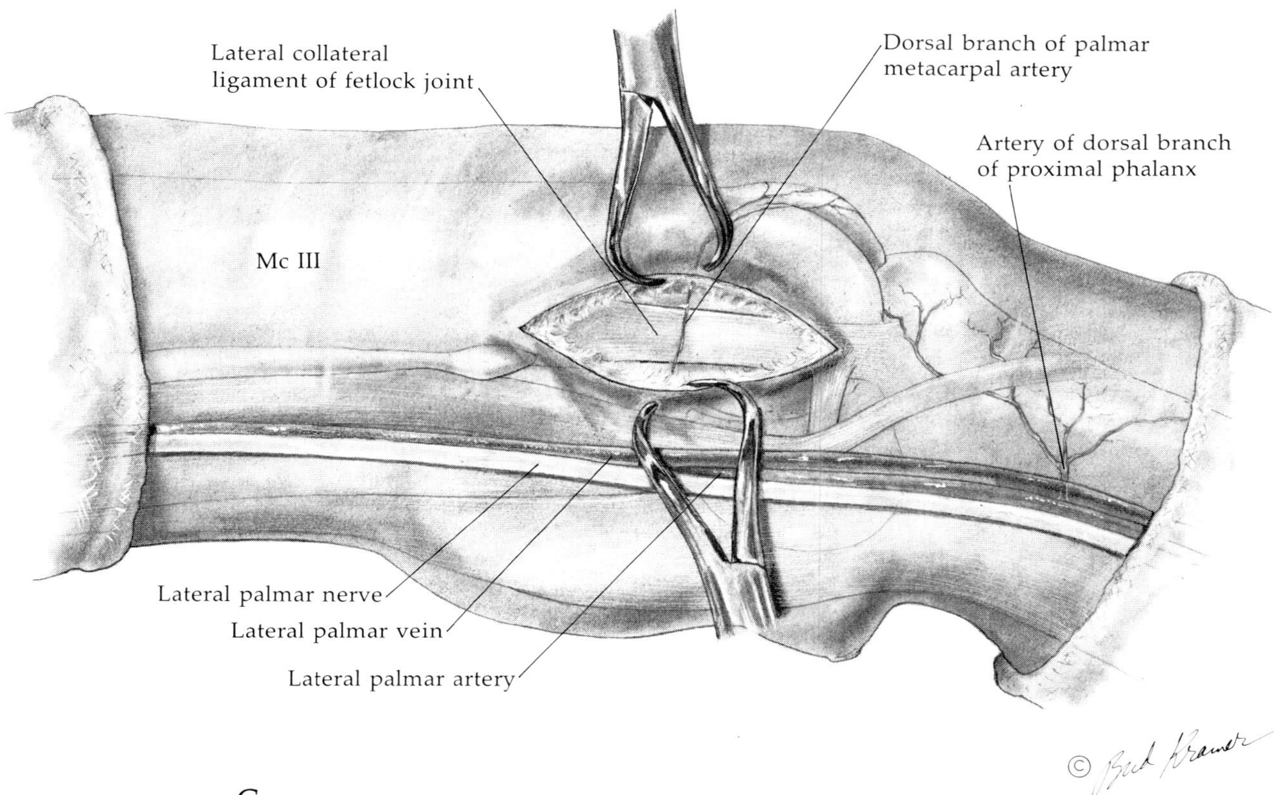

C

MEDIAL APPROACH TO THE THIRD METACARPUS (Mc III)

INDICATION

1. Open reduction and internal fixation of fractures of Mc III.[1–7]

POSITIONING OF PATIENT

The patient is placed with the affected limb down.

DESCRIPTION OF PROCEDURE

A. *Topographical View.* A curvilinear incision approximately 26 cm. long is made through the skin on the medial aspect of the Mc III, from the medial condyle of Mc III to the proximal-cranial aspect of Mc II.

B. *Surgeon's View.* The apex of the skin incision is directed caudally over the medial aspect of the interosseous (suspensory) ligament and deep digital flexor tendon. The base of the skin incision lies cranially over the cranial-medial aspect of the Mc III. The skin incision is made carefully, so as not to extend through the medial-dorsal metacarpal artery and vein where they cross the proximal-medial aspect of the metacarpus. The skin is reflected cranially from the apex of the incision toward the cranial-medial aspect of Mc III. A straight incision is made through the superficial fascia over the third metacarpal shaft, extending from the medial tuberosity of the metacarpus to the proximal-cranial aspect of the head of the second metacarpal bone. The medial-dorsal metacarpal artery and vein should be identified and preserved.

CLOSURE

The subcutaneous fascia is closed with an interrupted or continuous suture pattern. The skin should be closed with an interrupted suture pattern, with the incised edges in firm apposition.

COMMMENTS

The medial approach is used for fractures of the third metacarpus because the common digital extensor tendon lies laterally and it can be avoided with this approach. The metacarpus is basically axially loaded so that placing a bone plate on the medial or cranial-medial aspect of the bone is biomechanically sound.[7]

References

1. Alexander, J. T., and Rooney, R. J.: The Biomechanics, Surgery and Prognosis of Equine Fractures. *In* Proceedings, 18th Annual Meeting, American Association Equine Practitioners, 1972. (1973): 219–235.
2. Dingwall, J. S., Duncan, D. B., and Horney, F. D.: Compression Plating in Large Animal Orthopedics. J.A.V.M.A. *158* (1971): 1651–1657.
3. Fessler, J. F., and Amstutz, H. E.: *In* Oehme, F. W., and Prier, J. E. (eds.): Large Animal Surgery. Baltimore, the Williams & Wilkins Company, 1974, pp. 309–312.
4. Gertson, K. E., and Brinker, W. O.: Fracture Repair in Ponies Using Bone Plates. J.A.V.M.A. *154* (1969): 900–905.
5. Gertson, K. E., Monfort, J. N., and Tillotson, P. J. Fracture Repair in Large Animals. Vet. Med. Small Anim. Clin. *68* (1973): 782–790.
6. Milne, D. W., Turner, A. S., and Gabel, A. A. Surgical Approaches to Certain Long Bones of the Horse for Application of Tension Band Plates. J.A.V.M.A. *168* (January 1, 1976): 48–52.
7. Turner, A. S., Milne, D. W., and Gabel, A. A.: The Dynamic Compression Plate in Equine Long Bone Fractures. J.A.V.M.A. *168* (1976): 309–315.

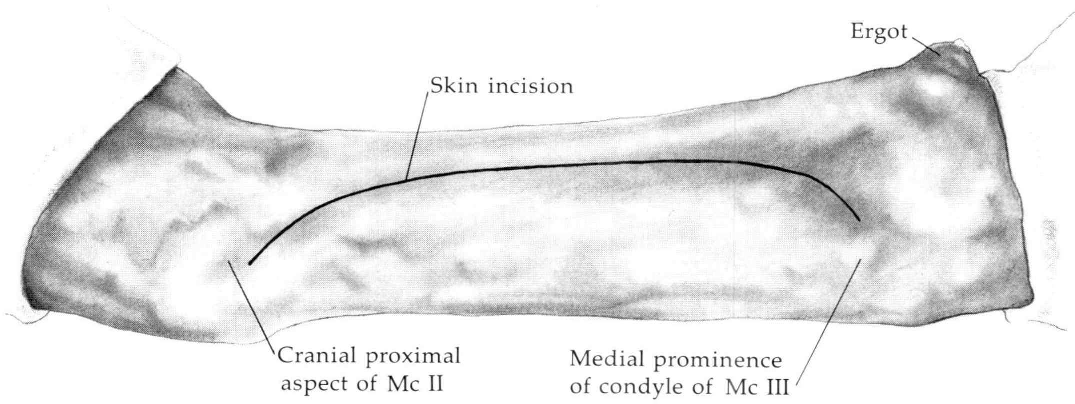
Ergot
Skin incision
Cranial proximal
aspect of Mc II
Medial prominence
of condyle of Mc III

A

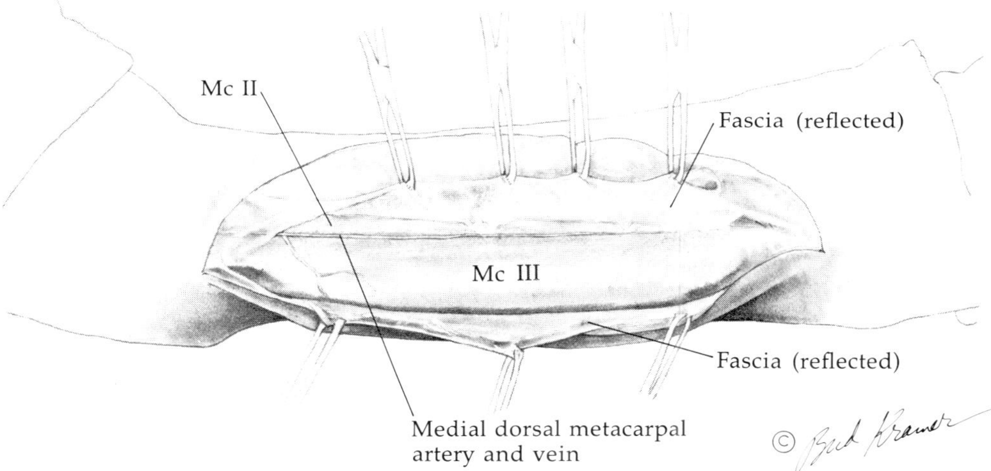
Mc II
Fascia (reflected)
Mc III
Fascia (reflected)
Medial dorsal metacarpal
artery and vein
© Bud Kramer

B

LATERAL APPROACH TO Mc II – MEDIAL SPLINT BONE

INDICATION

1. Surgical excision of the distal fragment of fractures of the second metacarpus, (Mc II).[1–5]
2. Surgical excision of bone sequestra involving Mc II.[1, 4]

POSITIONING OF PATIENT

The horse is positioned in right or left lateral recumbency with the affected limb down.

DESCRIPTION OF PROCEDURE

A. *Topographical View.* A variable length skin incision is made directly over the lateral aspect of Mc II, extending from approximately 1 cm. distal to the distal extremity of Mc II to approximately 2 cm. proximal to the proposed site of amputation.

B. *Surgeon's View.* The subcutaneous fascia is incised along the same line as the skin incision, extending to, but not through, the periosteum* covering Mc II. Once the skin and subcutaneous fascia are incised and retracted, Mc II should be immediately visible.

C. *Diagrammatic View of Tendons and Ligaments in Relationship to Bones.* When removing the distal portion of Mc II, care must be taken not to incise through the interosseous (suspensory) ligament lying caudal-medial to it. When dissecting the most distal portion of Mc II free from the surrounding fascia, the small interosseous (suspensory) tendon is incised or retracted as it passes over the distal extremity of Mc II.

---

*See Comments.

LATERAL APPROACH TO Mc II—MEDIAL SPLINT BONE

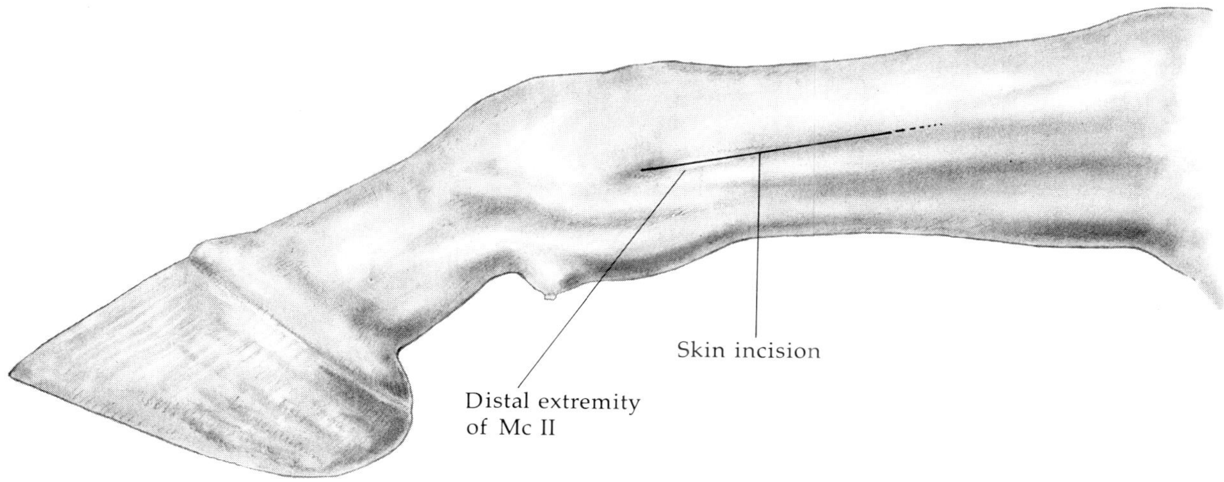

A

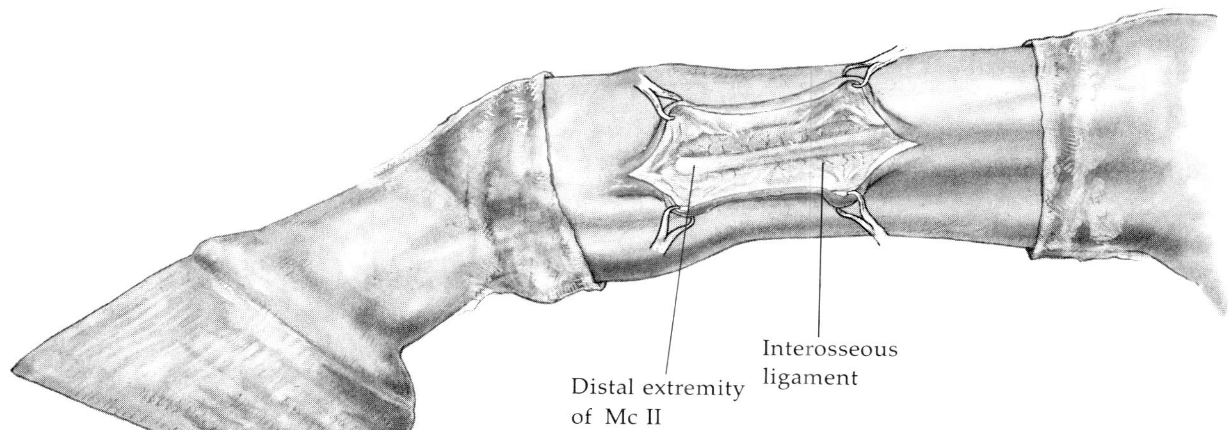

B

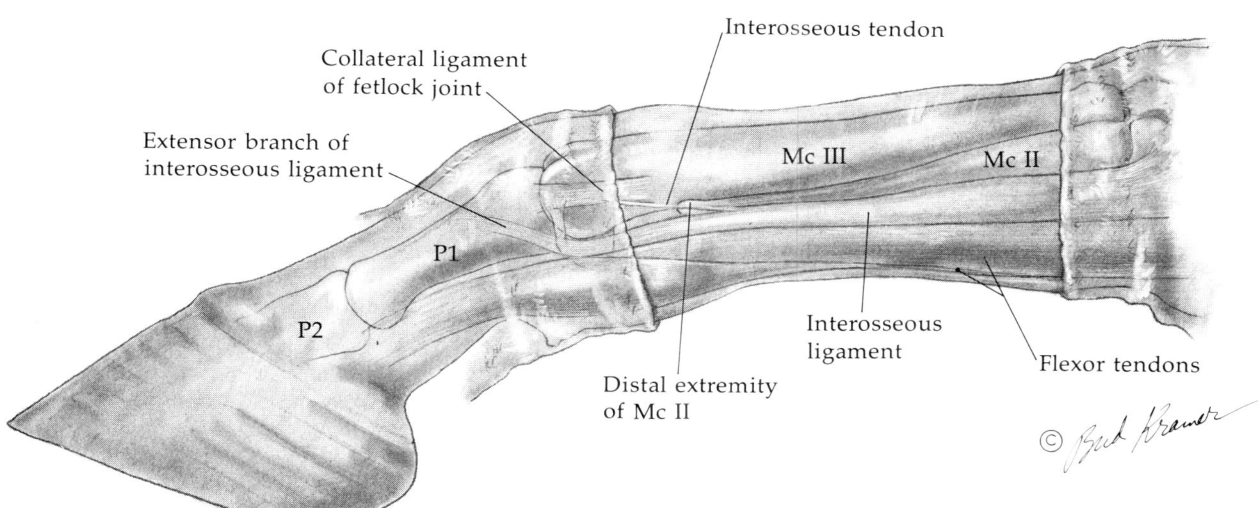

C

D. *Diagrammatic View of Vessels in Relationship to Tendons, Ligaments, and Bones.* The dorsal metacarpal artery II lies above and between Mc II and Mc III in the interosseous space. It can be ligated if necessary. The palmar metacarpal artery II lies deep, caudal and medial to Mc II and is largest at the level of the proximal third of Mc II. It supplies the nutrient artery to Mc III and continues distally as a small, more superficial artery. When amputating Mc II proximal to the junction of its upper and middle third, it should be identified and protected throughout the procedure.* The smaller, more superficial distal branch may be ligated if necessary. The medial palmar vein is far enough caudal to be out of the plane of dissection.

CLOSURE

An interrupted or continuous suture pattern can be used to close the subcutaneous fascia. The skin should be closed with an interrupted suture pattern with the incised edges in firm apposition.

COMMENTS

When excising the distal fragment of Mc II fractures, the surgeon may choose to dissect the bone out of its surrounding periosteum, and subsequently suture it closed after removal of the distal fragment.[1] This procedure is time consuming and does not appear to be necessary. It is recommended that the periosteum be removed along with the distal fragment.

When amputating proximal to the junction of the upper and middle third of Mc II, the surgical procedure becomes more difficult and dissection must be meticulous. The interosseous ligament lies deep in the metacarpal groove, closely associated with the caudal-medial aspect of Mc II. The interosseous ligament is difficult to retract at this level because it attaches to the proximal part of the caudal surface of Mc III and the distal row of carpal bones. In addition, palmar metacarpal artery II is large and must be preserved.

The lateral approaches to Mc II and Mc IV are essentially the same. The nutrient artery can originate from either the medial or lateral palmar metacarpal artery.[5] The approach to Mc II is described because these fractures are more common.[2]

*See Comments.

References

1. Adams, O. R.: Lameness in Horses. 3rd ed., Philadelphia, Lea and Febiger, 1974, pp. 210–213.
2. Jones, R. D., and Fessler, J. F.: Observations on Small Metacarpal and Metatarsal Fractures With or Without Associated Suspensory Desmitis in Standardbred Horses. Can. Vet. J. *18* (2) (1977): 29–32.
3. Numans, S. R., and Wintzer, H. J.: Surgical Treatment of Splint Bone Fractures. Tierarz. Wchschr. *74* (11) (1961): 205–210.
4. Rose, R. J.: Surgical Treatment of Osteomyelitis in the Metacarpal and Metatarsal Bones of the Horse. Vet. Rec. *102* (1978): 498–500.
5. Wintzer, H. J.: Fractures of Equine Small Metacarpal or Metatarsal Bones. Tierarz, Wchschr. *73* (13) (1960): 244.

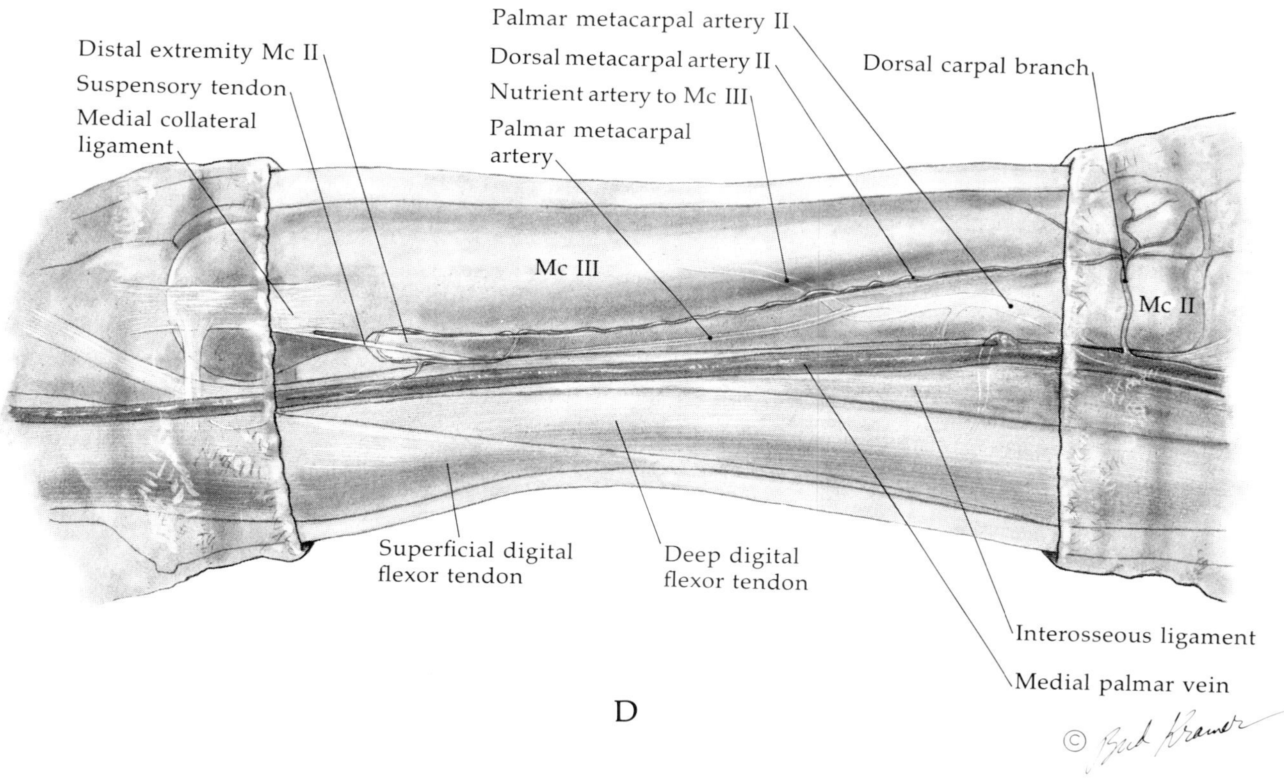
Palmar metacarpal artery II
Distal extremity Mc II
Dorsal metacarpal artery II
Dorsal carpal branch
Suspensory tendon
Nutrient artery to Mc III
Medial collateral ligament
Palmar metacarpal artery
Mc III
Mc II
Superficial digital flexor tendon
Deep digital flexor tendon
Interosseous ligament
Medial palmar vein
©

D

part six

Approaches to the Carpal Joint

CRANIAL-MEDIAL APPROACH TO DISTAL RADIOCARPAL BONE AND PROXIMAL THIRD CARPAL BONE (RADIAL FACET)

INDICATION

1. Surgical excision of chip fractures and osteophytes of the proximal third carpal bone and distal radiocarpal bone.[1, 2, 4–7]
2. Surgical curettage of ulcerative lesions of the medial aspect of the articular surfaces of the intercarpal joint.

POSITIONING OF PATIENT

The horse is positioned in right or left lateral recumbency with the affected limb down.

DESCRIPTION OF PROCEDURE

A. *Topographic View.* A curvilinear skin incision (base approximately 5 cm.), with the apex directed medially, is made over the cranial-medial aspect of the intercarpal joint, medial to the extensor carpi radialis tendon. The incision extends from the middle of the face of the radiocarpal bone to the middle of the face of the third carpal bone. The base of the skin incision should lie along the medial edge of the extensor carpi radialis tendon. The skin is reflected from the subcutaneous fascia toward the base.

B. *Surgeon's View.* A straight incision approximately 5 cm. long is made through the subcutaneous fascia, carpal annular ligament, and joint capsule, extending from approximately 1 cm. proximal to the distal border of the radiocarpal bone to approximately 1 cm. distal to the proximal border of the third carpal bone. This incision is made parallel to and approximately 1 cm. from the medial border of the tendon of the extensor carpi radialis muscle. Care should be taken to avoid incising its tendon sheath at the level of the distal end of the radiocarpal bone where the tendon sheath ends. The carpal joint is placed in flexion as the two edges of the joint capsule are retracted medially and laterally, exposing the articular surfaces of the intercarpal joint.

CRANIAL-MEDIAL APPROACH TO DISTAL RADIOCARPAL BONE AND PROXIMAL THIRD CARPAL BONE (RADIAL FACET)

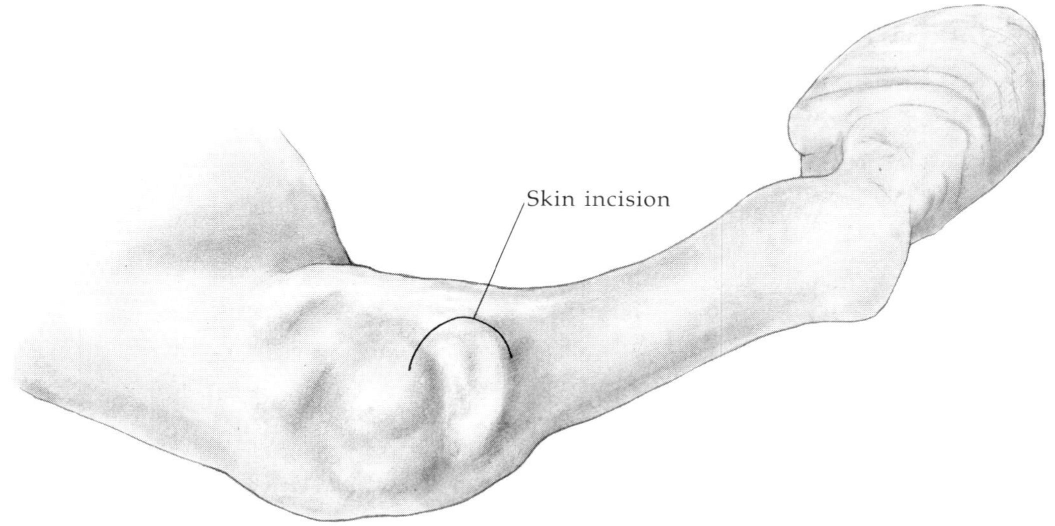

A

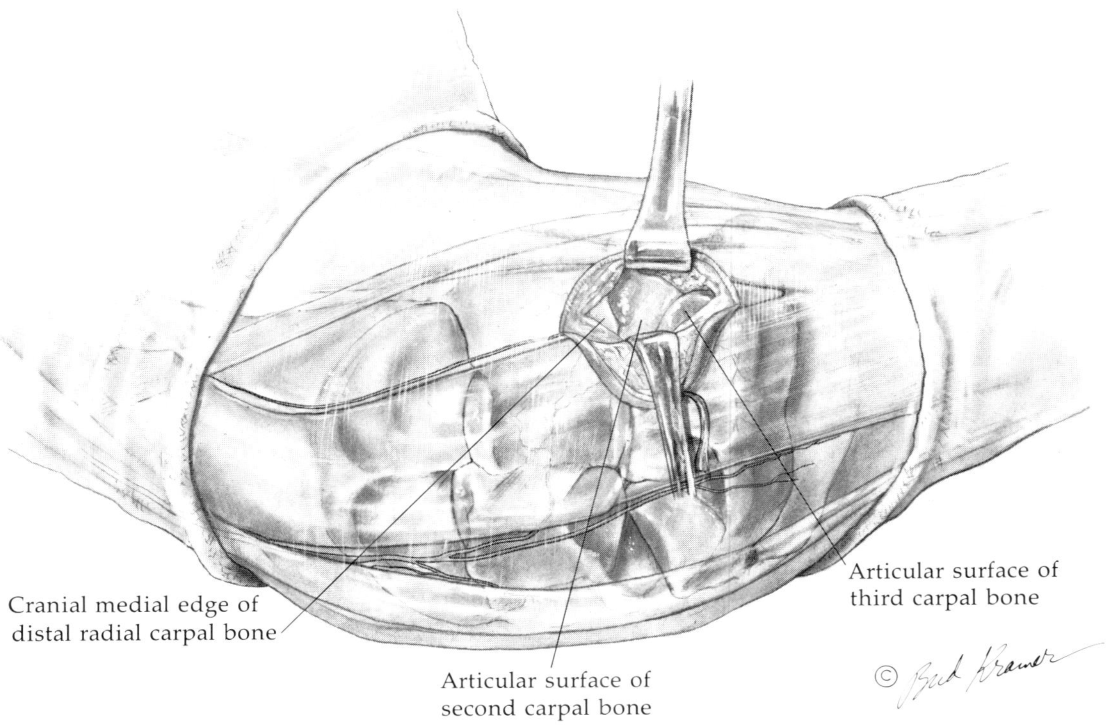

B

CRANIAL-MEDIAL APPROACH TO DISTAL RADIOCARPAL BONE AND PROXIMAL THIRD CARPAL BONE (RADIAL FACET)

C. *Diagrammatic View of Ligaments, Tendons, and Vessels Relative to Bones.* The approach to the intercarpal joint is centered between the lateral edge of the medial collateral ligament of the carpus and the medial edge of the extensor carpi radialis tendon. The branches of the cranial interosseous artery supply the joint capsule in this area. The transected branches of these arteries to the joint capsule should be carefully ligated.

D. *Surgeon's View.* A more cranial view of articular surfaces of the intercarpal joint. This view is more commonly seen when approaching fractures in the intercarpal joint.

CRANIAL-MEDIAL APPROACH TO DISTAL RADIOCARPAL BONE AND PROXIMAL THIRD CARPAL BONE (RADIAL FACET)

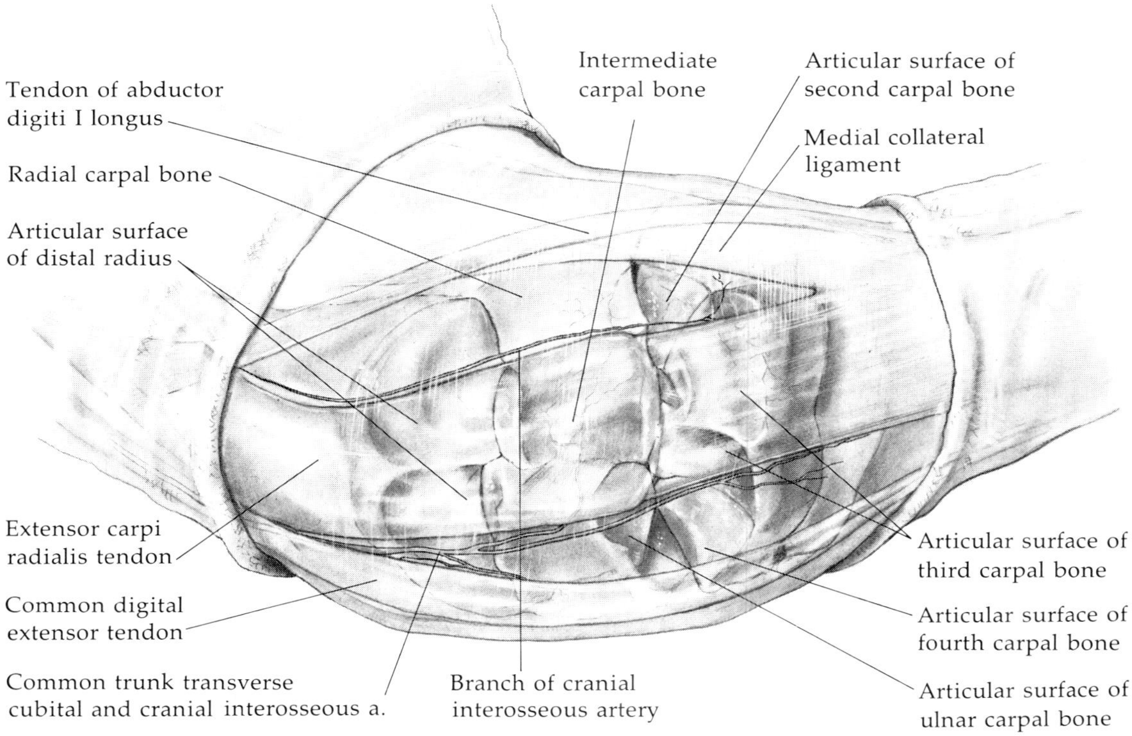

C

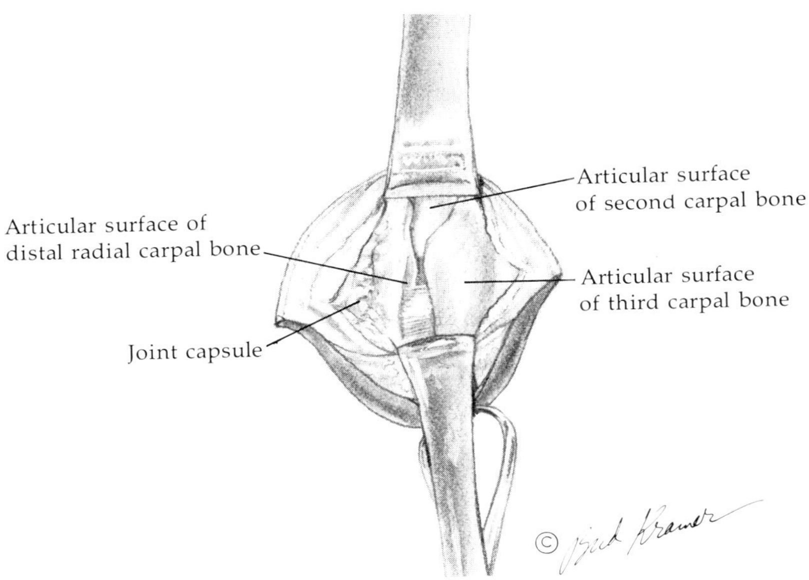

D

CLOSURE

The joint capsule (including the carpal annular ligament), subcutaneous fascia, and skin should be closed separately. The sutures in the joint capsule should not penetrate the synovial membrane; the synovial membrane of the joint capsule should not be allowed to evert between the apposed edges of the fibrous joint capsule, as this reduces the rate and strength of healing.[3] Preplacement of the sutures in the joint capsule will allow a more accurate approximation of the cut edges of the joint capsule and achieve a tight seal (each suture is tied after all the sutures have been placed). An interrupted suture pattern is recommended for closure of the joint capsule. An interrupted or continuous suture pattern can be used to close the subcutaneous fascia. The skin should be closed with an interrupted suture pattern so that the incised edges are in firm apposition.

COMMENTS

The cranial-medial aspects of the distal radiocarpal bone and proximal aspect of the third carpal bone are the most common sites for chip fractures in the carpus of the horse.[5, 6, 7] Consequently, this is a common surgical approach.

A straight incision may be utilized in the skin along the same line as the incision through the subcutaneous fascia, carpal annular ligament, and joint capsule. The advantage of the curvilinear incision is that the location of the medial border of the extensor carpi radialis is more easily discernible once the skin is reflected from the subcutaneous fascia. This allows the surgeon to make the incision in the annular ligament and joint capsule with more precision. In addition, the curvilinear incision is easily extended in the skin to obtain a more cranial exposure to the joint.

Visualization of the articular surfaces of the cranial-medial aspect of the intercarpal joint is aided by: 1) retraction of the joint capsule; 2) altering the position of the carpus with regards to different degrees of flexion. When replacing or removing retractors in the joint, the carpus should be placed in extension. This relaxes the joint capsule and the extensor carpi radialis tendon. Relaxing these structures allows easier placement and removal of retractors, minimizing trauma to the articular surfaces of the carpal bones.

References

1. Adams, O. R.: Lameness in Horses. 3rd ed., Philadelphia, Lea and Febiger, 1974, pp. 187–195.
2. Heinze, C. D.: Equine Orthopedic Surgery. Mod. Vet. Prac. (Red Book), (Oct. 15, 1966): 63–84.
3. International Symposium of Sutures in Wound Repair. London, England, Ethicon, U.S.A. July, 1972.
4. Larson, L. H., and Dixon, R. T.: Management of Carpal Injuries in the Fast Gaited Horse. Aust. Vet. J. *46* (1970): 133–139.
5. Park, R. D., Morgan, J. P., and O'Brien, T. R.: Chip Fractures in the Carpus of the Horse: A Radiographic Study of Their Incidence and Location. J.A.V.M.A. *157* (10) (1970): 1306–1311.
6. Thrall, E. D., Lebel, J. L., and O'Brien, T. R.: A Five Year Survey of the Incidence and Location of Equine Carpal Chip Fractures. J.A.V.M.A. *158* (1971): 1366–1368.
7. Wyburn, R. S., and Goulden, B. E.: Fractures of the Equine Carpus: A Report of 57 Cases. New Zealand Vet. J. *22* (1974): 133–142.

CRANIAL-MEDIAL APPROACH TO THE CRANIAL-MEDIAL ASPECT OF THE THIRD CARPAL BONE

INDICATIONS

1. Open reduction of slab fractures of the third carpal bone.[1, 2, 4-7]
2. Surgical removal of slab fractures of the third carpal bone.

POSITIONING OF PATIENT

The horse is positioned in right or left lateral recumbency with the affected limb down.

DESCRIPTION OF PROCEDURE

A. *Topographical View.* A curvilinear skin incision (base approximately 6 cm.), with the apex directed medially, is made over the cranial-medial aspect of the intercarpal joint, medial to the extensor carpi radialis tendon. The incision extends from the middle of the face of the radiocarpal bone to the carpometacarpal joint. The base of the skin incision should be along the medial edge of the extensor carpi radialis tendon. The skin is reflected from the subcutaneous fascia toward the base.

B. *Surgeon's View.* A straight incision approximately 5 cm. long is made through the subcutaneous fascia, carpal annular ligament, and joint capsule, extending from approximately 1 cm. proximal to the distal border of the radiocarpal bone to approximately 1 cm. proximal to the distal border of the third carpal bone. This incision is made parallel to and approximately 1 cm. from the medial border of the extensor carpi radialis tendon. Care should be taken to avoid incising its tendon sheath at the level of the distal end of the radiocarpal bone where the tendon sheath ends. The carpal joint is placed in flexion as the two edges of the joint capsule are retracted medially and laterally, exposing the articular surface of the intercarpal joint and the cranial face of the third carpal bone.

CRANIAL-MEDIAL APPROACH TO THE CRANIAL-MEDIAL ASPECT OF THE THIRD CARPAL BONE

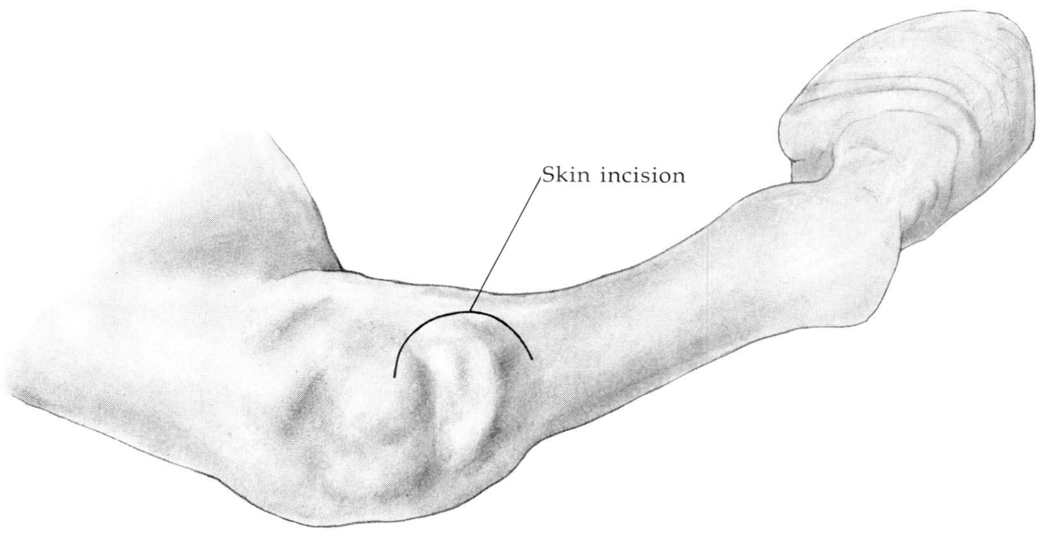

A

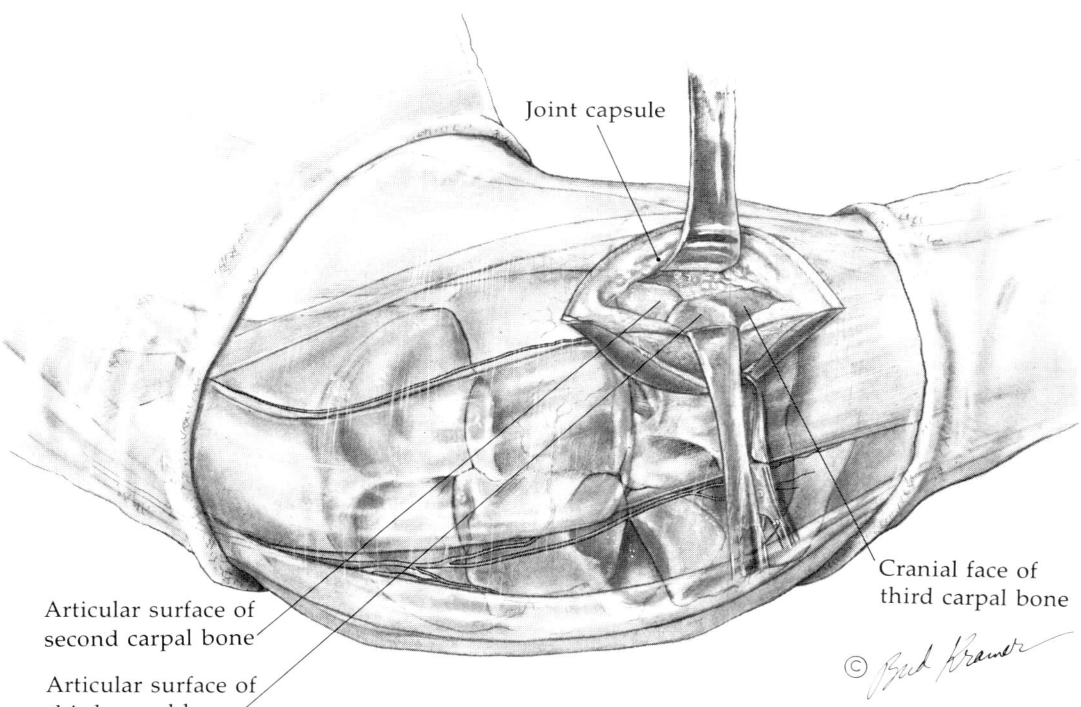

B

CRANIAL-MEDIAL APPROACH TO CRANIAL-MEDIAL ASPECT OF THIRD CARPAL BONE

C. *Diagrammatic View of Ligaments, Tendons and Vessels Relative to Bones.* The incision in the joint capsule over the intercarpal joint is centered between the lateral edge of the medial collateral ligament of the carpus and the medial edge of the extensor carpi radialis tendon. The branches of the cranial interosseous artery supply the joint capsule in this area. The transected branches of these arteries in the joint capsule should be carefully ligated.

D. *Surgeon's View.* A more cranial view of articular surfaces of the intercarpal joint and cranial surface of the third carpal bone. This view is more commonly seen when approaching the cranial face of the third carpal bone.

CRANIAL-MEDIAL APPROACH TO THE CRANIAL-MEDIAL ASPECT OF THE THIRD CARPAL BONE

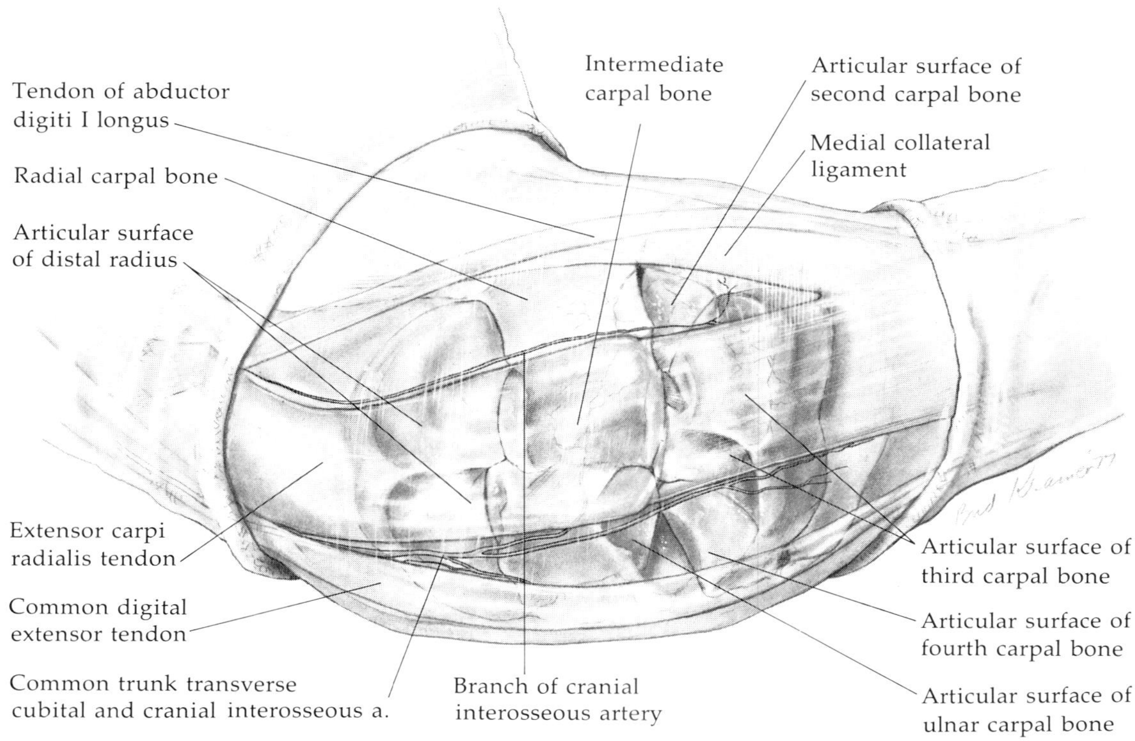

C

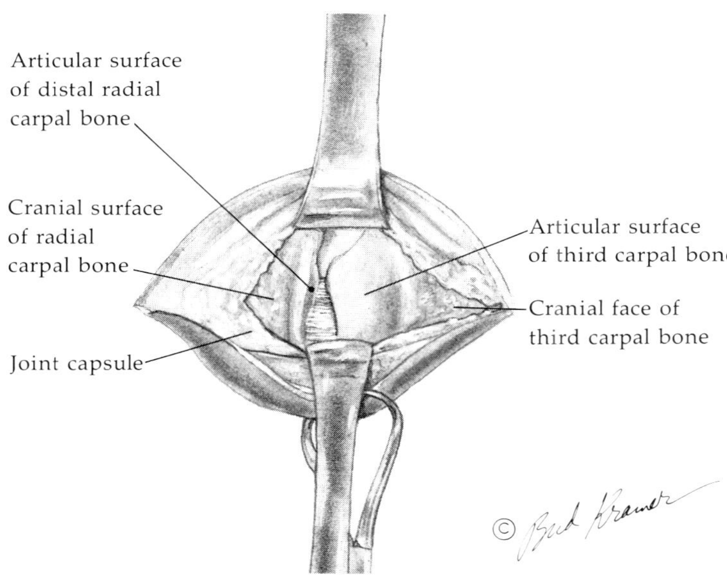

D

CRANIAL-MEDIAL APPROACH TO THE CRANIAL-MEDIAL ASPECT OF THE THIRD CARPAL BONE

CLOSURE

The joint capsule (including the carpal annular ligament), subcutaneous fascia, and skin should be closed separately. The sutures in the joint capsule should not penetrate the synovial membrane; the synovial membrane of the joint capsule should not be allowed to evert between the apposed edges of the fibrous joint capsule, as this reduces the rate and strength of healing.[3] Preplacement of the sutures in the joint capsule will allow a more accurate approximation of the cut edges of the joint capsule and achieve a tight seal (each suture is tied after all the sutures have been placed). An interrupted suture pattern is recommended for closure of the joint capsule. An interrupted or continuous suture pattern can be used to close the subcutaneous fascia. The skin should be closed with an interrupted suture pattern so that the edges are in firm apposition.

COMMENTS

The third carpal bone is the most common site for slab fractures in the carpus of the horse.[1, 2, 4-9] Consequently, this is a common surgical approach.

A straight incision may be utilized in the skin along the same line as the incision through the subcutaneous fascia, carpal annular ligaments, and joint capsule. The advantage of the curvilinear incision is that the location of the medial border of the extensor carpi radialis is more easily discernible once the skin is reflected from the subcutaneous fascia. This allows the surgeon to place the incision in the annular ligament and joint capsule with more precision. In addition, the curvilinear incision is easily extended in the skin to obtain a more cranial exposure in the annular ligament and joint capsule.

Visualization of the articular surfaces of the cranial medial aspect of the intercarpal joint is aided by: 1) retraction of the joint capsule; 2) altering the position of the carpus with regards to different degrees of flexion. When replacing or removing retractors in the joint, the carpus should be placed in extension. This relaxes the joint capsule and extensor carpi radialis tendon. Relaxing these structures allows easier placement and removal of retractors, minimizing trauma to the articular surfaces of the carpal bones.

This approach enables accurate alignment of the articular surface at the fracture site and is recommended over a simple stab incision on the cranial face of the third carpal bone for placement of a screw. Opening the intercarpal joint also enables the surgeon to remove osteochondral fragments that frequently occur along the fracture site at the articular surface.

In some cases, the slab fracture will be located in such a manner that the center of the slab lies beneath the extensor carpi radialis tendon where it passes over the cranial face of the third carpal bone. In these cases, the skin flap is extended and reflected more craniolaterally, so that a stab incision can be made through the extensor carpi radialis tendon and joint capsule for placement of an interfragmentary screw at the cranial face of the third carpal bone.

CRANIAL-MEDIAL APPROACH TO THE CRANIAL-MEDIAL ASPECT OF THE THIRD CARPAL BONE

References

1. Adams, O. R.: Lameness in Horses. 3rd ed., Philadelphia, Lea and Febiger, 1974, pp. 187–195.
2. Heinze, C. D.: Equine Orthopedic Surgery. Mod. Vet. Pract. (Red Book) (October 15, 1966): 63–84.
3. International Symposium of Sutures in Wound Repair. London, England, Ethicon, U.S.A. July, 1972.
4. Larson, L. H. and Dixon, R. T.: Management of Carpal Injuries in the Fast Gaited Horse. Aust. Vet. J. *46* (1970): 33–39.
5. Manning, J. P., and St. Clair, L. E.: Surgical Repair of the Third Carpal Bone Fractures in the Thoroughbred Horse. Illinois Vet. *3* (1960): 106–111.
6. Park, R. D., Morgan, J. P., and O'Brien, T. R.: Chip Fractures in the Carpus of the Horse: A Radiographic Study of their Incidence and Location. J.A.V.M.A. *157* (10) (1970): 1306–1311.
7. Raker, C. W. Orthopedic Surgery: Errors in Surgical Evaluation and Management. *In* Proceedings, 19th Annual Meeting, American Association Equine Practitioners, 1973. (1974): 206.
8. Thrall, E. D., Lebel, J. L., and O'Brien, T. R.: A Five Year Survey of the Incidence and Location of Equine Carpal Chip Fractures. J.A.V.M.A. *158* (1971): 1366–1368.
9. Wyburn, R. S., and Goulden, B. E.: Fractures of the Equine Carpus: A Report of 57 Cases. New Zealand Vet. J. *22* (1974): 133–142.

CRANIAL-MEDIAL APPROACH TO THE DISTAL RADIUS AND PROXIMAL RADIOCARPAL BONE

INDICATIONS

1. Surgical excision of chip fractures and osteophytes of the distal radius and proximal radiocarpal bone.[1, 2, 4–7]
2. Surgical curettage of ulcerative lesions of the medial aspect of the articular surfaces of the radiocarpal joint.

POSITIONING OF THE PATIENT

The horse is positioned in right or left lateral recumbency with the affected limb down.

DESCRIPTION OF PROCEDURE

A. Topographic View. A curvilinear skin incision (base approximately 5 cm.) with the apex directed medially is made over the cranial-medial aspect of the radiocarpal joint medial to the extensor carpi radialis tendon and lateral to the tendon of abductor digiti I longus (extensor carpi obliquus). The incision extends from approximately 1 cm. proximal to the distal radius to the middle of the face of the radiocarpal bone. The base of the skin incision should lie along the medial edge of the extensor carpi radialis tendon. The skin is reflected from the subcutaneous fascia toward the base.

B. Surgeon's View. A straight incision approximately 5 cm. long is made through the subcutaneous fascia, carpal annular ligament, and joint capsule extending from approximately 1 cm. proximal to the distal border of the radius to the middle of the face of the radiocarpal bone. The incision is made parallel to and 1 cm. from the medial border of the tendon of the extensor carpi radialis muscle. Care should be taken to avoid incising its tendon sheath. The carpal joint is placed in flexion as the two edges of the joint capsule are retracted medially and laterally, exposing the articular surfaces of the radiocarpal joint.

CRANIAL-MEDIAL APPROACH TO THE DISTAL RADIUS AND PROXIMAL RADIOCARPAL BONE

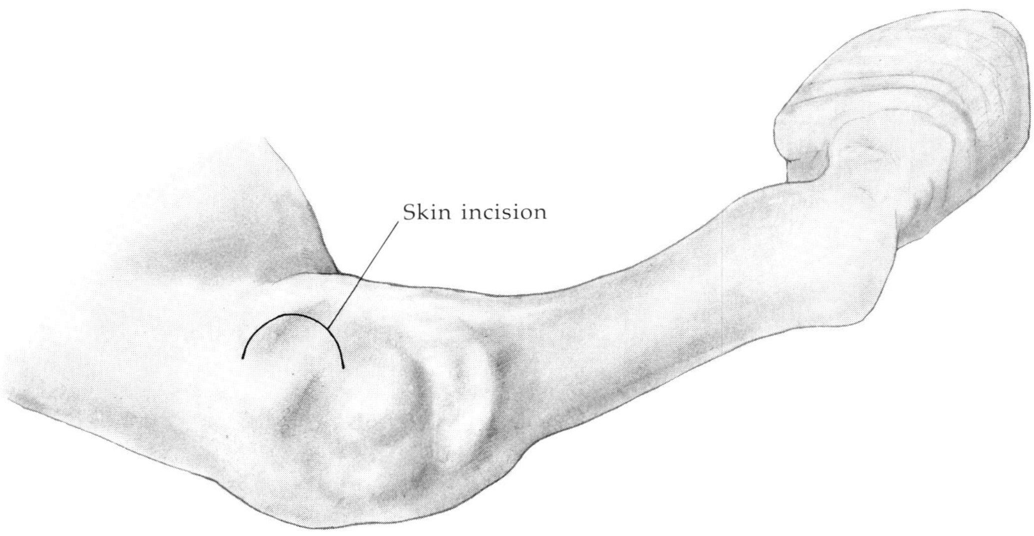

A

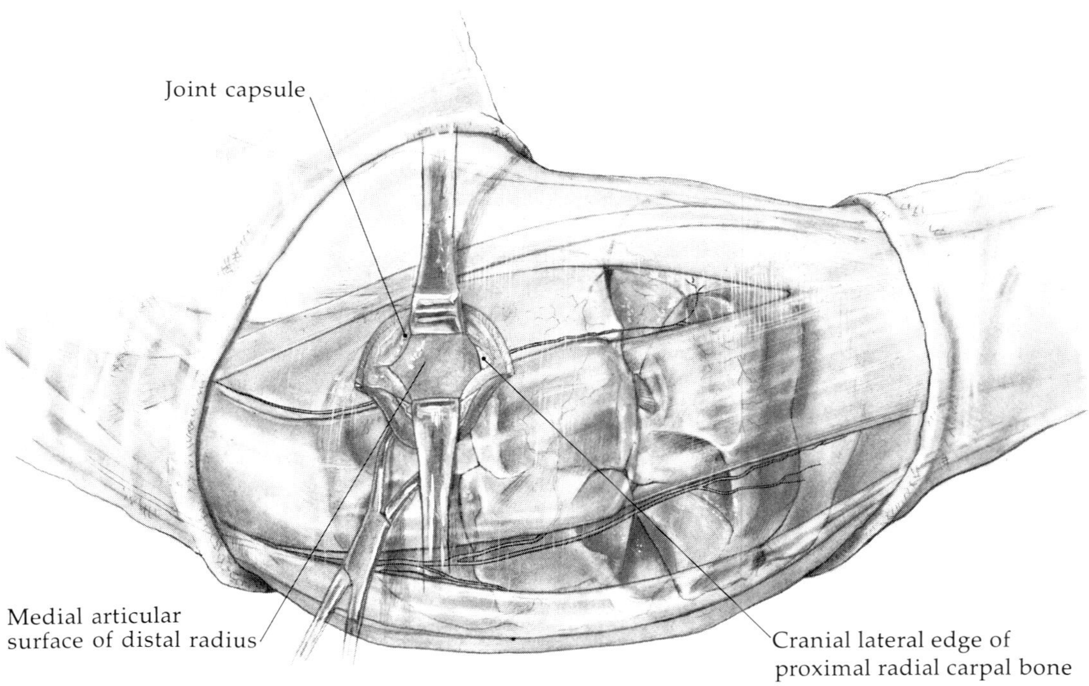

B

C. *Diagrammatic View of Ligaments, Tendons, and Vessels Relative to Bones.* The approach to the radiocarpal joint is centered between the lateral border of the tendon of the abductor digiti I longus (extensor carpi obliquus) and the medial edge of the extensor carpi radialis tendon. The branches of the cranial interosseous artery supply the joint capsule in this area. The transected branches of these arteries in the joint capsule should be carefully ligated.

D. *Surgeon's View.* A more cranial view of the articular surfaces of the radiocarpal joint is seen more commonly when approaching fractures of the radiocarpal joint.

CLOSURE

The joint capsule (including carpal annular ligament) subcutaneous tissues, and skin should be closed separately. The sutures in the joint capsule should not penetrate the synovial membrane; the synovial membrane of the joint capsule should not be allowed to evert between the opposed edges of the fibrous joint capsule, as this reduces the rate and strength of healing.[3] Preplacement of the sutures in the joint capsule will allow a more accurate approximation of the cut edges of the joint capsule and achieve a tight seal (each suture is tied after all the sutures have been placed). An interrupted pattern should be used for closure of the joint capsule. An interrupted or continuous pattern can be used to close the subcutaneous fascia. The skin should be closed with an interrupted pattern so that the incised edges are in firm apposition.

COMMENTS

Fractures of the cranial-medial aspect of the distal radius are considerably less common than fractures of the cranial-lateral aspect of the distal radius.[5-7]

A straight incision may be utilized in the skin along the same line as the incision through the subcutaneous fascia, carpal annular ligament, and joint capsule. The advantage of the curvilinear incision is that the location of the medial border of the extensor carpi radialis tendon is more easily discernible once the skin is reflected from the subcutaneous fascia. This allows the surgeon to make the incision in the annular ligament and joint capsule with more precision. In addition, the curvilinear incision in the skin is easily extended to obtain a more cranial exposure.

Visualization of the articular surfaces of the cranial-medial aspect of the radiocarpal joint is aided by: 1) retraction of the joint capsule; 2) altering the position of the carpus with regards to different degrees of flexion. When inserting or removing retractors in the joint, the carpus should be placed in extension. This relaxes the joint capsule and the extensor carpi radialis tendon. Relaxing these structures allows easier placement and removal of retractors, minimizing trauma to the articular surfaces of the carpal bones.

References

1. Adams, O. R.: Lameness in Horses. 3rd ed., Philadelphia, Lea and Febiger, 1974, pp. 187–195.
2. Heinze, C. D.: Equine Orthopedic Surgery. Mod. Vet. Pract. (Red Book) October 15, 1966: 63–84.
3. International Symposium of Sutures in Wound Repair. London, England, Ethicon, U.S.A. July, 1972.
4. Larson, L. H., and Dixon, R. T.: Management of Carpal Injuries in the Fast Gaited Horse. Australian Vet. J. *46*: (1970): 133–139.
5. Park, R. D., Morgan, J. P., and O'Brien, T. R.: Chip Fractures in the Carpus of the Horse: A Radiographic Study of Their Incidence and Location. J.A.V.M.A. *157* (10) (1970): 1306–1311.
6. Thrall, E. D., Lebel, J. L., and O'Brien, T. R.: A Five Year Survey of the Incidence and Location of Equine Carpal Chip Fractures. J.A.V.M.A. *158* (1971): 1366–1368.
7. Wyburn, R. S., and Goulden, B. E.: Fractures of the Equine Carpus: A Report of 57 Cases. New Zealand Vet. J. *22* (1974): 133–142.

CRANIAL-MEDIAL APPROACH TO THE DISTAL RADIUS AND PROXIMAL RADIOCARPAL BONE

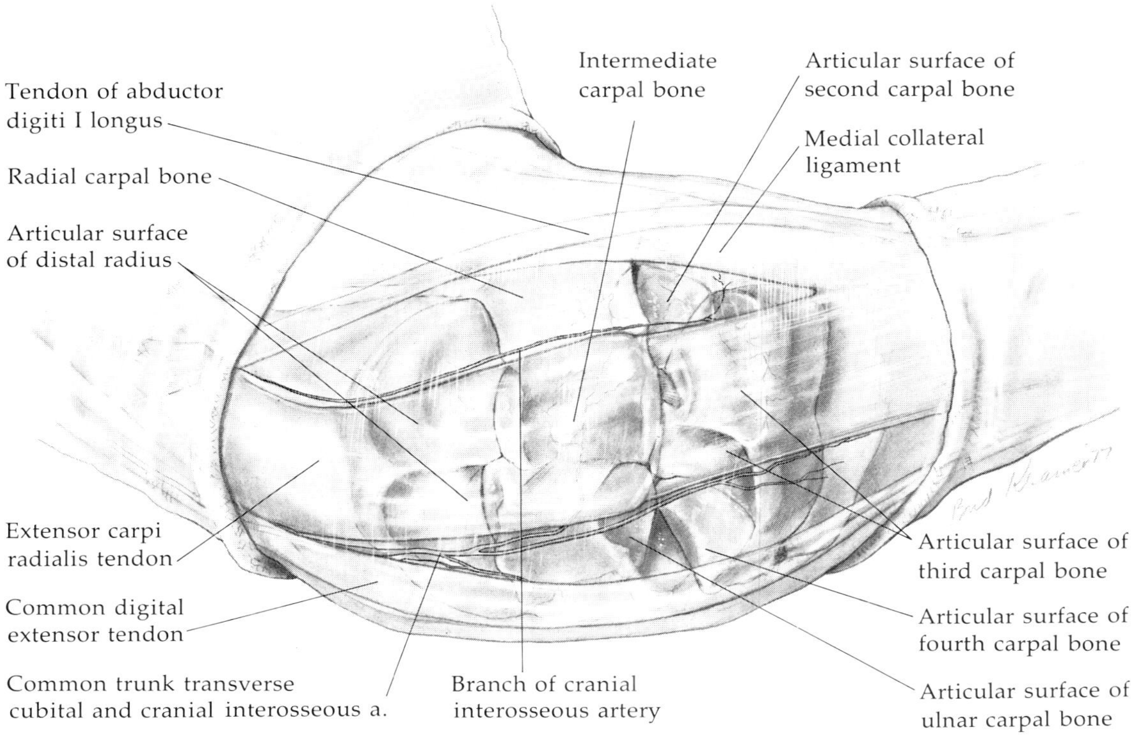

C

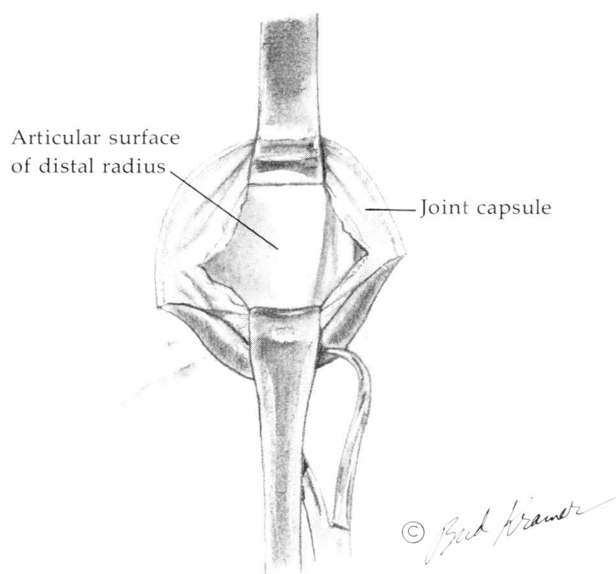

D

CRANIAL-LATERAL APPROACH TO PROXIMAL THIRD CARPAL BONE (INTERMEDIATE FACET) AND DISTAL INTERMEDIATE CARPAL BONE

INDICATIONS

1. Surgical excision of chip fractures and osteophytes of the proximal third carpal bone and distal intermediate carpal bone.[1, 2, 4-7]
2. Surgical curettage of ulcerative lesions of the cranial-lateral articular surfaces of the intercarpal joint.

POSITIONING OF THE PATIENT

The horse is positioned in right or left lateral recumbency with the affected limb uppermost.

DESCRIPTION OF THE PROCEDURE

A. *Topographical View.* A curvilinear skin incision (base approximately 5 cm. long) with the apex directed laterally is made over the cranial-lateral aspect of the intercarpal joint, lateral to the extensor carpi radialis tendon and medial to the common digital extensor tendon. The incision extends from the middle of the face of the intermediate carpal bone to the middle of the face of the third carpal bone. The base of the skin incision should lie along the lateral edge of the extensor carpi radialis tendon. The skin is reflected from the subcutaneous fascia toward the base.

B. *Surgeon's View.* A straight incision approximately 5 cm. long is made through the subcutaneous fascia, carpal annular ligament, and joint capsule, extending from approximately 1 cm. proximal to the distal border of the intermediate carpal bone to approximately 1 cm. distal to the proximal border of the third carpal bone. This incision is made midway between the extensor carpi radialis tendon and the common digital extensor tendon. Care should be taken to avoid incising the tendon sheaths of either of these tendons. The carpal joint is placed in flexion as the two edges of the joint capsule are retracted medially and laterally, exposing the articular surfaces of the intercarpal joint.

CRANIAL-LATERAL APPROACH TO PROXIMAL THIRD CARPAL BONE (INTERMEDIATE FACET) AND DISTAL INTERMEDIATE CARPAL BONE

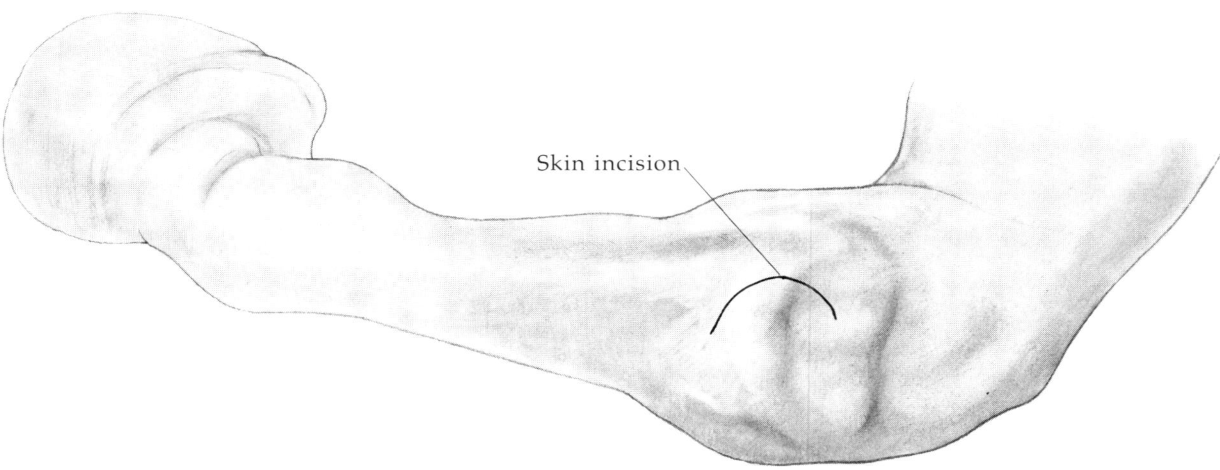

A

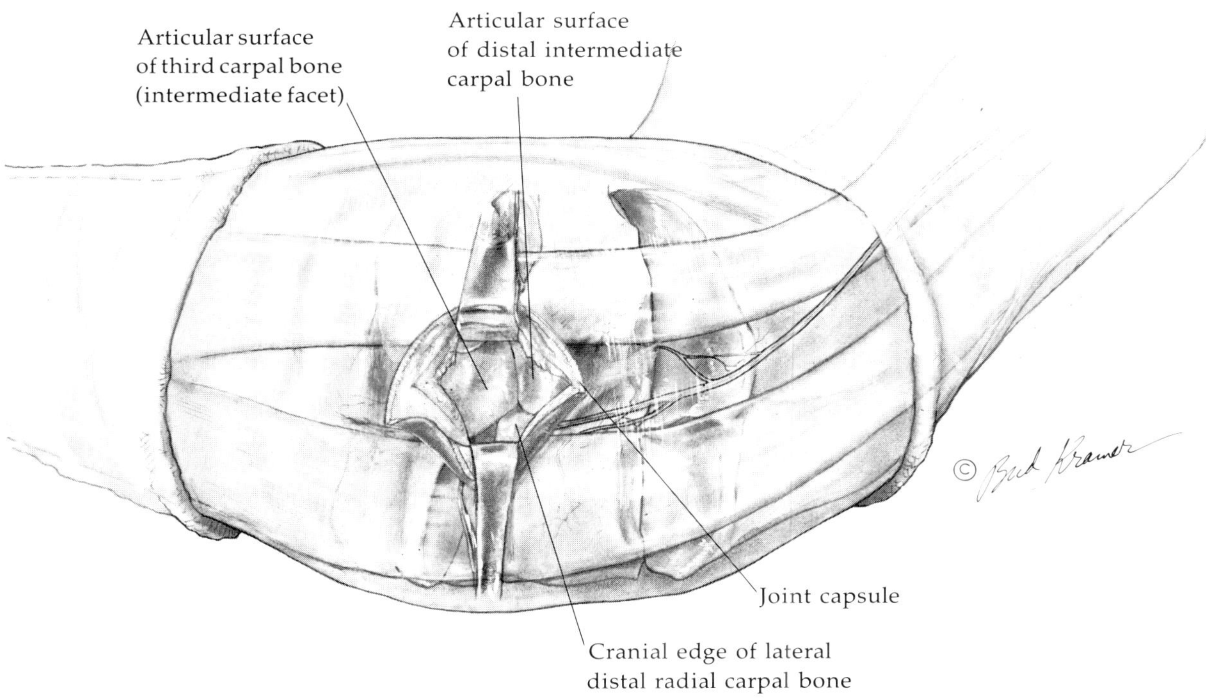

B

C. Diagrammatic View of Ligaments, Tendons and Vessels Relative to Bones. This approach to the intercarpal joint is centered between the lateral edge of the extensor carpi radialis tendon and the common digital extensor tendon. The branches of the common trunk of the cranial interosseous and the transverse cubital arteries supply the joint capsule in this area. The transected branches of these arteries to the joint capsule should be carefully ligated.

CLOSURE

The joint capsule (including the carpal annular ligament), subcutaneous tissues, and skin should be closed separately. The sutures in the joint capsule should not penetrate the synovial membrane, nor should the synovial membrane be allowed to evert between the opposed edges of the fibrous joint capsule.[3] Preplacement of the sutures in the joint capsule will allow a more accurate approximation of the cut edges of the joint capsule and achieve a tight seal (each suture is tied after all sutures have been placed). Interrupted patterns are recommended for closure of the joint capsule. An interrupted or continuous pattern can be used to close the subcutaneous fascia. The skin should be closed with an interrupted pattern so that the wound edges are in firm apposition.

COMMENTS

Fractures of the cranial-lateral aspect of the proximal third carpal bone (intermediate facet) and the opposing surface of the distal intermediate carpal bone are considerably less common than fractures of the distal radiocarpal bone and opposing surface of the third carpal bone (radial facet).[5-7]

A straight incision may be utilized in the skin along the same line as the incision through the subcutaneous fascia, carpal annular ligament, and joint capsule. The advantage of the curvilinear incision is that the locations of the lateral border of the extensor carpi radialis and the medial border of the common digital extensor tendon are more easily discernible once the skin incision is reflected from the subcutaneous fascia. This allows the surgeon to make the incision in the annular ligament and joint capsule with more precision. In addition, the curvilinear incision is easily extended in the skin to obtain a more cranial exposure in the carpal annular ligament and joint capsule.

Visualization of the articular surfaces of the cranial-lateral aspect of the intercarpal joint is aided by: 1) retraction of the joint capsule; 2) altering the position of the carpus with regard to differing degrees of flexion. When inserting or removing retractors in the joint, the carpus should be placed in extension. This relaxes the joint capsule and the extensor carpi radialis tendon. Relaxing these structures allows easier placement and removal of the retractors, minimizing trauma to the articular surfaces of the carpal bones.

CRANIAL-LATERAL APPROACH TO PROXIMAL THIRD CARPAL BONE (INTERMEDIATE FACET) AND DISTAL INTERMEDIATE CARPAL BONE

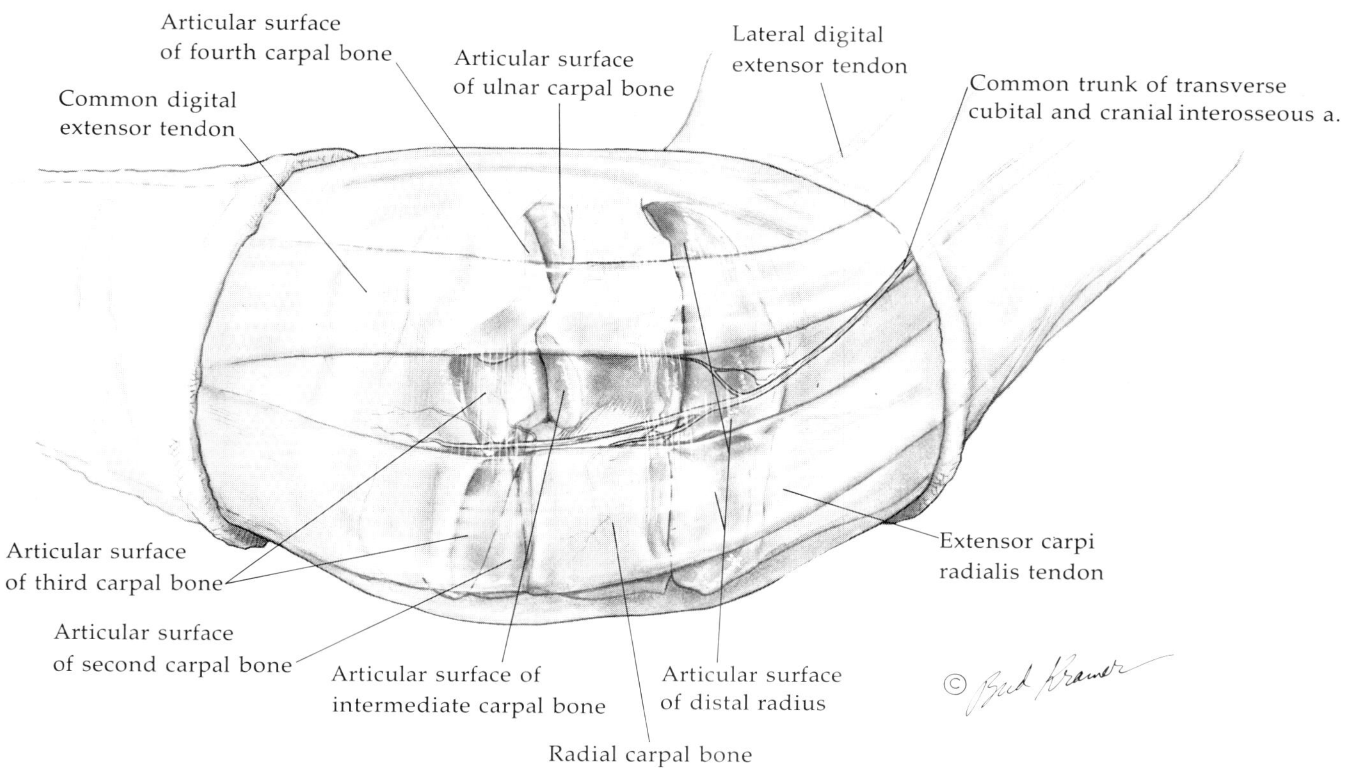

C

References

1. Adams, O. R.: Lameness in Horses. 3rd ed., Philadelphia, Lea and Febiger, 1974, pp. 187–195.
2. Heinze, C. D.: Equine Orthopedic Surgery. Mod. Vet. Pract. (Red Book) (Oct., 1966): 63–84.
3. International Symposium of Sutures in Wound Repair. London, England, Ethicon U.S.A. July, 1972.
4. Larson, L. H., and Dixon, R. T.: Management of Carpal Injuries in the Fast Gaited Horse. Aust. Vet. J. *46* (Feb. 1970):133–139.
5. Park, R. D., Morgan, J. P., and O'Brien, T. R.: Chip Fractures in the Carpus of the Horse: A Radiographic Study of Their Incidence and Location. J.A.V.M.A. *157* (10) (1970):1306–1311.
6. Thrall, E. D., Lebel, J. L., and O'Brien, T. R.: A Five Year Survey of the Incidence and Location of Equine Carpal Chip Fractures. J.A.V.M.A. *158* (1971):1366–1368.
7. Wyburn, R. S., and Goulden, B. E.: Fractures of the Equine Carpus: A Report of 57 Cases. New Zealand Vet. J. *22* (1974):133–142.

CRANIAL-LATERAL APPROACH TO DISTAL RADIUS, PROXIMAL RADIAL CARPAL BONE, AND PROXIMAL INTERMEDIATE CARPAL BONE.

INDICATIONS

1. Surgical excision of chip fractures and osteophytes of the distal radius, proximal radial carpal bone and proximal intermediate carpal bone.[1, 2, 4-7]
2. Surgical curettage of ulcerative lesions of the cranial-lateral articular surfaces of the radiocarpal joint.

POSITIONING OF PATIENT

The horse is positioned in right or left lateral recumbency with the affected limb uppermost.

DESCRIPTION OF PROCEDURE

A. *Topographical View.* A curvilinear skin incision (base approximately 5 cm. long) with the apex directed laterally is made over the cranial-lateral aspect of the radiocarpal joint, lateral to the extensor carpi radialis tendon and medial to the common digital extensor tendon. The incision extends from approximately 1 cm. proximal to the distal radius to the level of the middle of the face of the radiocarpal bone. The base of the skin incision should lie along the lateral border of the extensor carpi radialis tendon.

B. *Surgeon's View.* A straight incision approximately 5 cm. long is made through the subcutaneous fascia, carpal annular ligament, and joint capsule extending from approximately 1 cm. proximal to the distal border of the radius to the level of the middle of the face of the radiocarpal bone.

CRANIAL-LATERAL APPROACH TO DISTAL RADIUS, PROXIMAL RADIAL CARPAL BONE, AND PROXIMAL INTERMEDIATE CARPAL BONE.

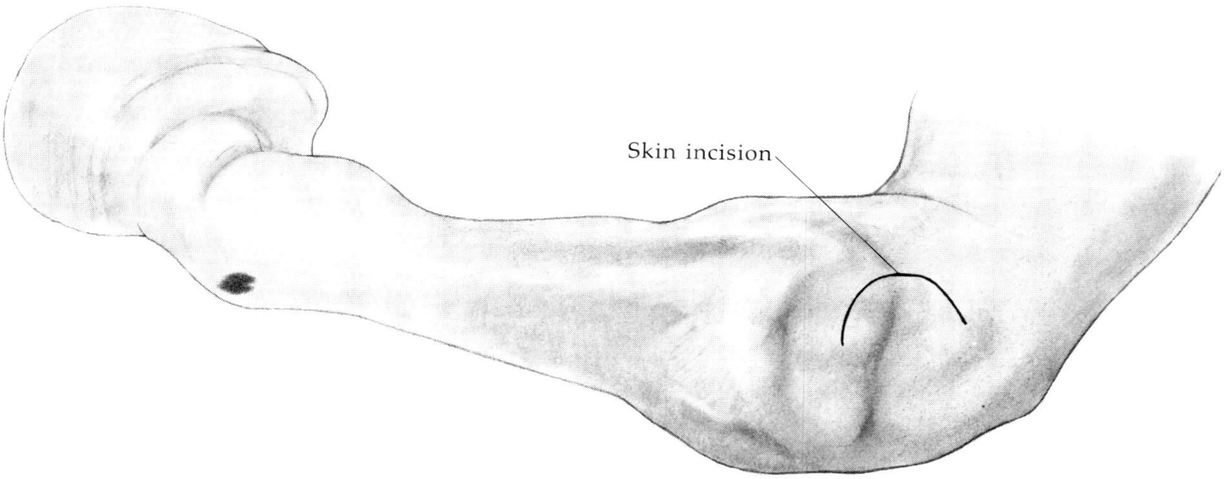

A

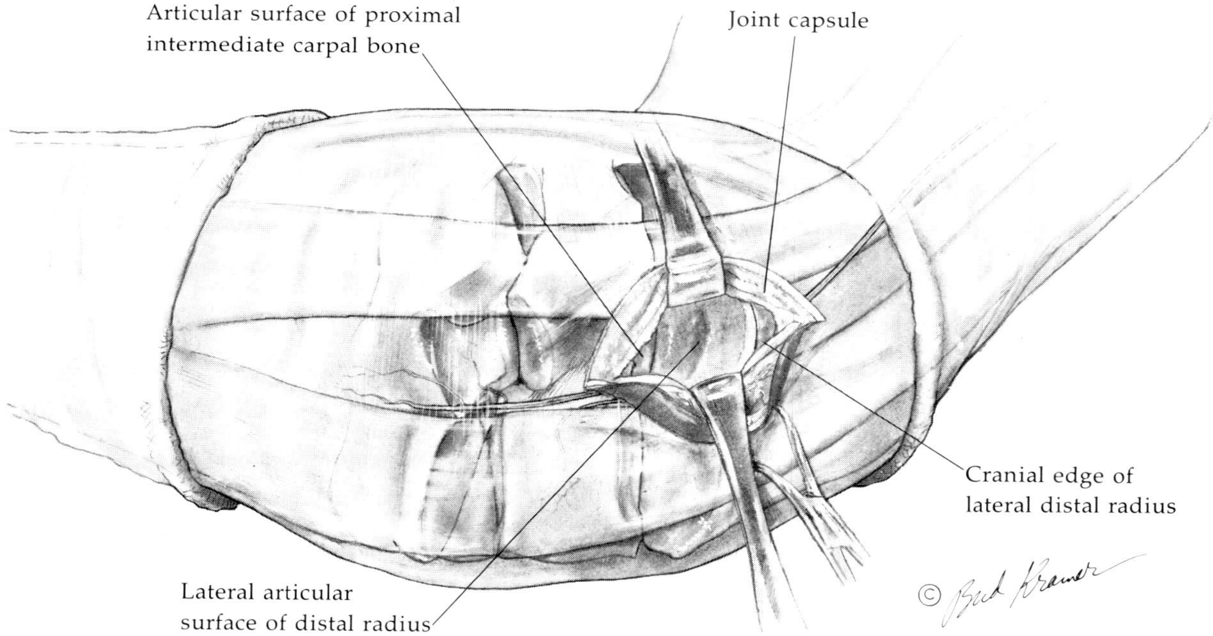

B

CRANIAL-LATERAL APPROACH TO DISTAL RADIUS, PROXIMAL RADIAL CARPAL BONE, AND PROXIMAL INTERMEDIATE CARPAL BONE.

C. Diagrammatic View of Ligaments, Tendons and Vessels Relative to the Bones. The approach to the radiocarpal joint is centered between the lateral border of the extensor carpi radialis tendon and the medial border of the common digital extensor tendon. The branches of the common trunk for the cranial interosseous and transverse cubital arteries supply the joint capsule in this area. The transected branches of these arteries to the joint capsule should be carefully ligated.

CLOSURE

The joint capsule (including the carpal annular ligament), subcutaneous tissues, and skin should be closed separately. The sutures in the joint capsule should not penetrate the synovial membrane; the synovial membrane of the joint capsule should not be allowed to evert between the opposed edges of the fibrous joint capsule, as this reduces the rate and strength of healing.[3] Preplacement of the sutures in the joint capsule will allow a more accurate approximation of the cut edges of the joint capsule and achieve a tight seal (each suture is tied after all the sutures have been placed). Interrupted patterns are recommended for closure of the joint capsule. An interrupted or continuous pattern can be used to close the subcutaneous fascia. The skin should be closed with an interrupted pattern so that the incised edges are in firm apposition.

COMMENTS

Fractures of the cranial-lateral aspect of the distal radius are relatively common compared with fractures of the cranial-medial aspect.[5-7] Consequently this is a common surgical approach. A straight incision may be utilized in the skin along the same line as the incision through the subcutaneous fascia, carpal annular ligament, and joint capsule. The advantage of the curvilinear incision is that the locations of the lateral border of the extensor carpi radialis and the medial border of the common digital extensor tendon are more easily discernible once the skin is reflected from the subcutaneous fascia. This allows the surgeon to make the incision in the annular ligament and joint capsule with more precision. In addition, the curvilinear incision is easily extended to obtain a more cranial exposure in the carpal annular ligament and joint capsule.

Visualization of the articular surfaces of the cranial-lateral aspect of the radiocarpal joint is aided by: 1) retraction of the joint capsule; 2) altering the position of the carpus with regard to different degrees of flexion. When replacing retractors in the joint or removing them, the carpus should be placed in extension. This relaxes the joint capsule and the extensor carpi radialis tendon. Relaxing these structures allows easier placement and removal of retractors, minimizing trauma to the articular surfaces of the carpal bones.

References

1. Adams, O. R.: Lameness in Horses. 3rd ed., Philadelphia, Lea and Febiger, 1974, pp. 187–195.
2. Heinze, C. D.: Equine Orthopedic Surgery. Mod. Vet. Pract. (Red Book) (Oct. 15, 1966):63–84.
3. International Symposium of Sutures in Wound Repair. London, England, Ethicon, U.S.A. July, 1972.
4. Larson, L. H., and Dixon, R. T.: Management of Carpal Injuries in the Fast Gaited Horse. Aust. Vet. J. *46* (Feb. 1970):133–139.
5. Park, R. D., Morgan, J. P. and O'Brien, T. R.: Chip Fractures in the Carpus of the Horse: A Radiographic Study of Their Incidence and Location. J.A.V.M.A. *157* (10) (1970):1306–1311.
6. Thrall, E. D., Lebel, J. L., and O'Brien, T. R.: A Five Year Survey of the Incidence and Location of Equine Carpal Chip Fractures. J.A.V.M.A. *158* (1971):1366–1368.
7. Wyburn, R. S., and Goulden, B. E. Fractures of the Equine Carpus: A Report of 57 Cases. New Zealand Vet. J. *22* (1974):133–142.

CRANIAL-LATERAL APPROACH TO DISTAL RADIUS, PROXIMAL RADIAL CARPAL BONE, AND PROXIMAL INTERMEDIATE CARPAL BONE.

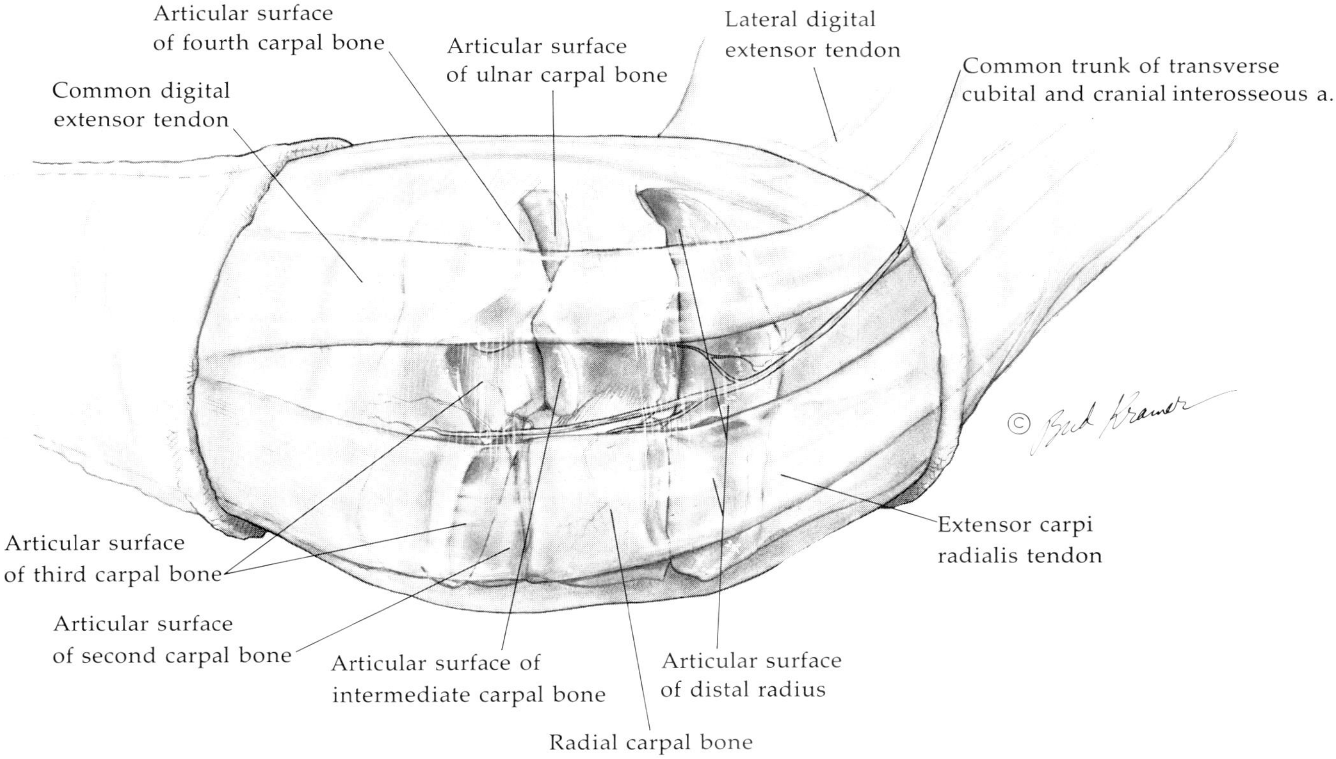

C

part seven

Approach to the Ulna and Olecranon

APPROACH TO THE CAUDAL AND LATERAL ASPECT OF THE ULNA AND OLECRANON

INDICATION

1. Surgical repair of fractures of the ulna and olecranon.[1-8]

POSITIONING OF PATIENT

The horse is positioned in right or left lateral recumbency with the affected limb uppermost.

DESCRIPTION OF PROCEDURE

A. *Topographical View.* A curvilinear skin incision approximately 26 cm. long is begun from a point approximately 2 cm. proximal to the attachment of the triceps tendon on the proximal aspect of the olecranon. The incision arcs over the lateral aspect of the olecranon and extends down the caudal-lateral aspect of the ulna, in the depression formed by the fascial planes between the ulnaris lateralis muscle and the ulnar head of the deep digital flexor muscle. Distally, the skin incision is made over the fascial planes between the ulnaris lateralis muscle and the tendon of the ulnar head of the deep digital flexor muscle.

B. *Surgeon's View.* The skin is reflected from the apex of the incision over the olecranon toward the caudal-lateral aspect of the ulna. When reflecting the skin, one will observe a cutaneous branch of the caudal cutaneous antebrachial nerve on the caudal aspect of the ulna, coursing distolaterally between the ulnar head of the deep digital flexor muscle and the caudal superficial pectoral muscle. It then comes to lie over the caudal-lateral aspect of the superficial digital flexor muscle. This nerve should be preserved. The subcutaneous incision is made from the point of the olecranon, along the depression formed by the fascial planes between the ulnaris lateralis muscle and the ulnar head of the deep digital flexor muscle.

APPROACH TO THE CAUDAL AND LATERAL ASPECT OF THE ULNA AND OLECRANON

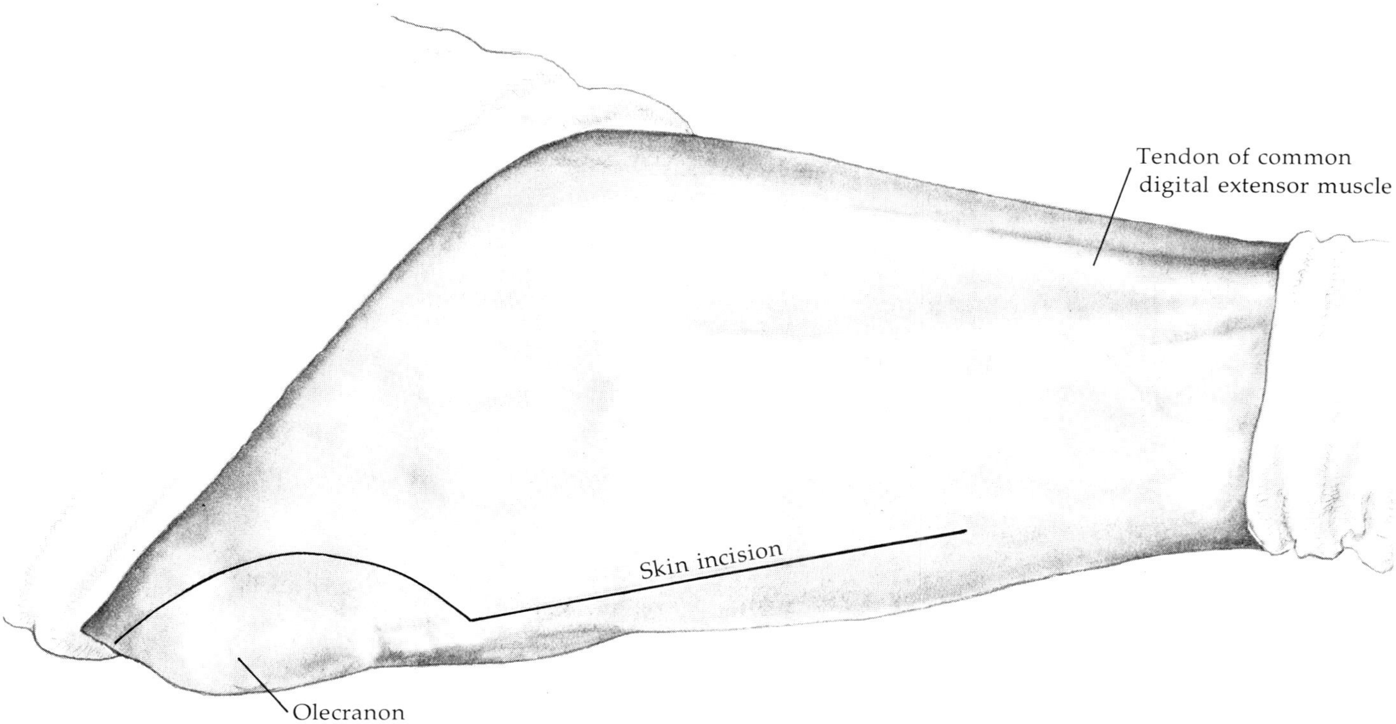

A

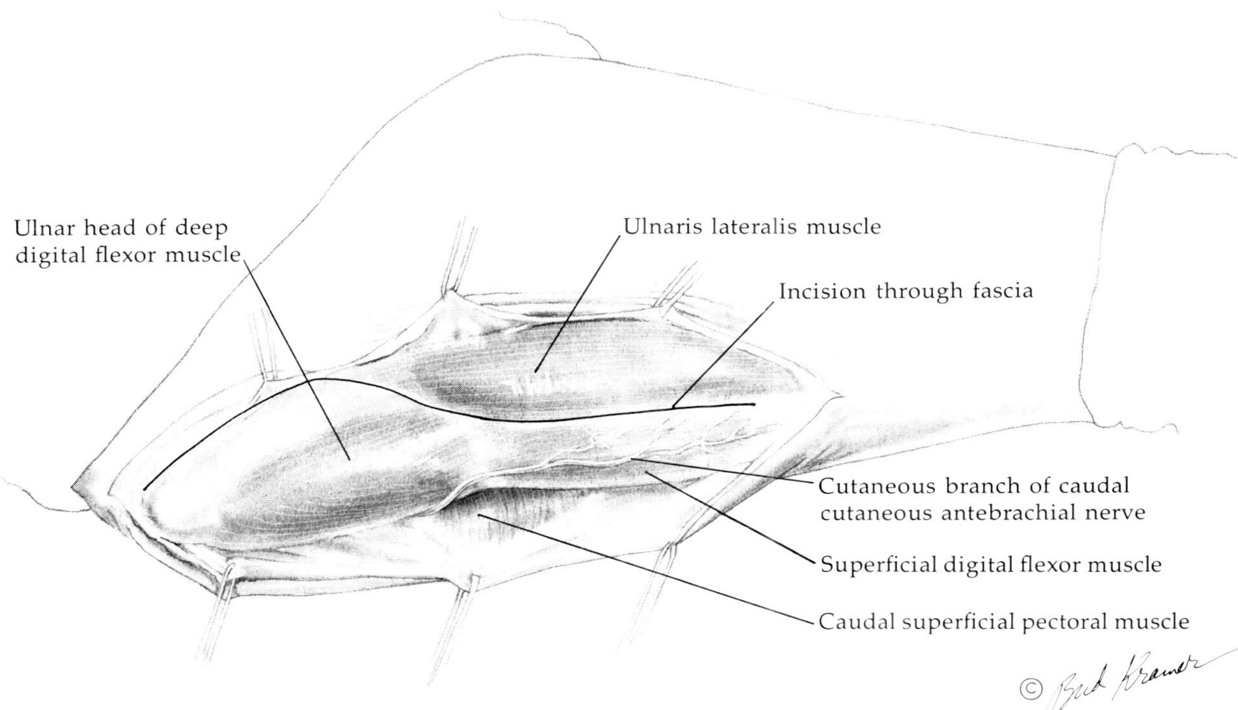

B

C. *Surgeon's View.* The incision is then extended deep through the fascial septum between the ulnaris lateralis muscle and ulnar head of the deep digital flexor muscle and tendon. At the level of the distal third of the ulna, the ulnar head of the deep digital flexor muscle becomes tendinous. As the ulnar nerve courses distally, it becomes superficial and lies just caudal to this tendon. It should be carefully preserved. The ulnaris lateralis muscle is reflected cranially and the ulnar head of the deep digital flexor caudally, exposing the caudal-lateral aspect of the ulna. To obtain better exposure of the caudal aspect of the ulna, the humeral head of the deep digital flexor muscle can be bluntly reflected from the caudal-medial aspect of the ulna.

D. *Surgeon's View (lateral approach).* To apply a plate to the lateral aspect of the ulna, further exposure may be required. The superficial fascia is reflected cranially to expose the fascial septum between the ulnaris lateralis and lateral digital extensor muscles. An incision is made through the intermuscular septum. The ulnaris lateralis muscle is reflected caudally and the lateral digital extensor muscle cranially, exposing the lateral aspect of the ulna. The muscular branches of the anastomotic loop formed by the cranial interosseous artery and vein, and branches of the transverse cubital artery and vein, as well as a muscular branch of the radial nerve, cross the septum between the ulnaris lateralis and lateral digital extensor muscles at the level of the distal third of the ulna (artery, nerve, and vein, from proximal to distal). These structures must be preserved.

APPROACH TO THE CAUDAL AND LATERAL ASPECT OF THE ULNA AND OLECRANON

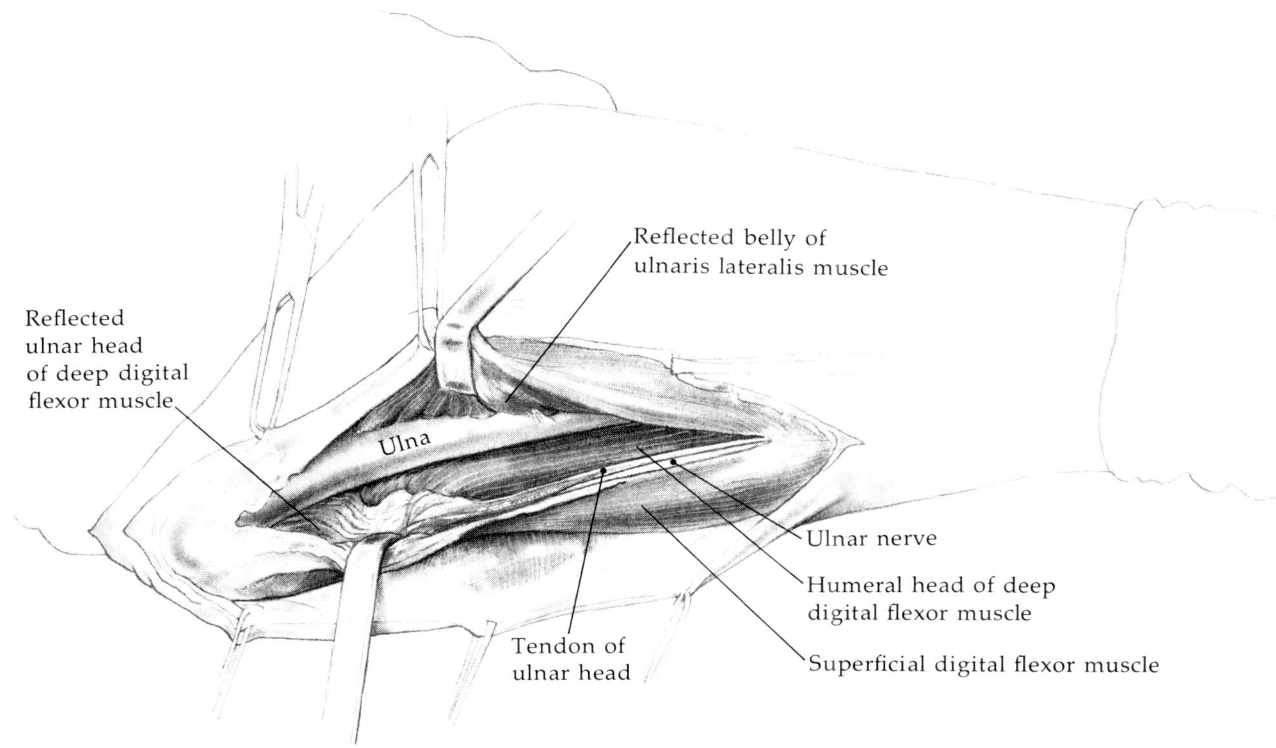

C

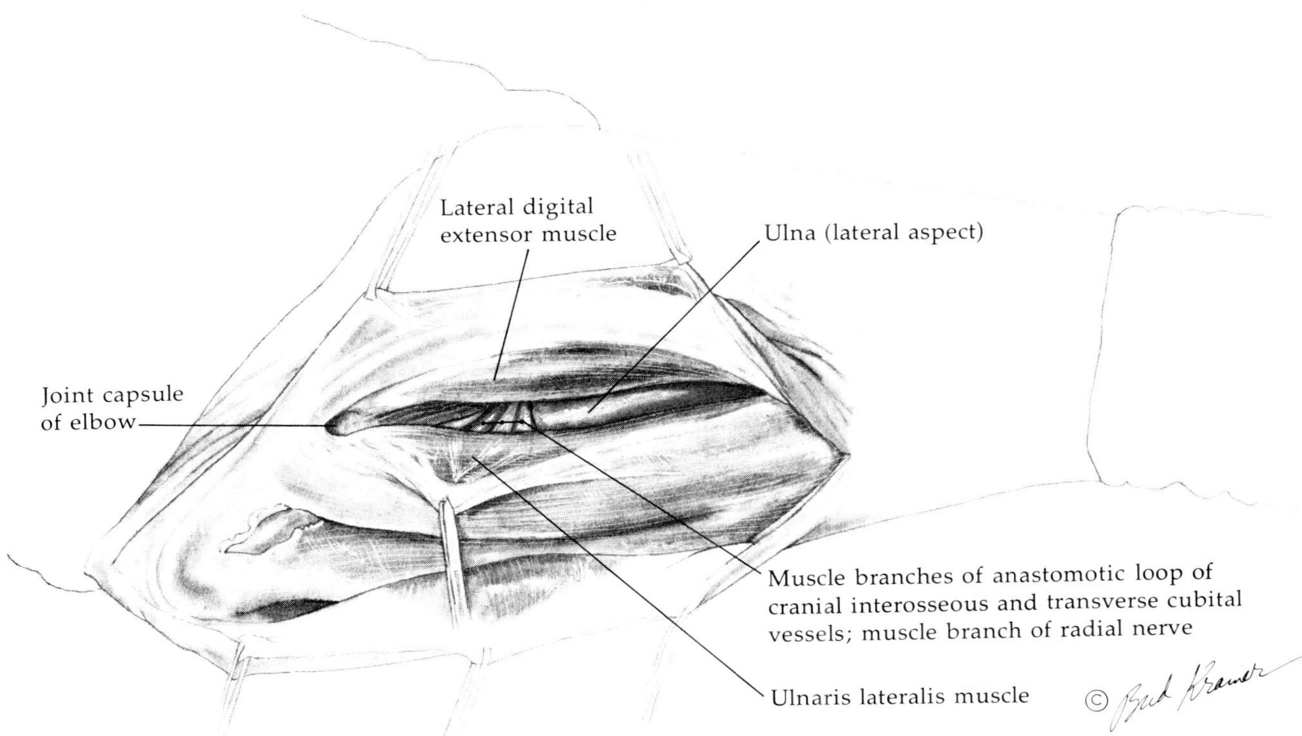

D

CLOSURE

The fascial planes between the ulnaris lateralis muscle and the ulnar head of the deep digital flexor muscle are closed using an interrupted or continuous pattern. The skin is closed using an interrupted pattern with the incised edges in firm apposition.

COMMENTS

The approach described is for the application of tension band plates to the caudal and lateral aspects of the ulna. Because of the pull of the triceps brachii muscle on the olecranon, the tension side of the ulna is the caudal aspect; therefore, the plate is usually applied on the caudal aspect. A plate may have to be applied to the lateral aspect of the ulna to reduce olecranon fractures at the elbow joint when the proximal fragment is severely distracted. The plate must be placed under the vessels and nerve encountered in the lateral approach. If the ulnaris lateralis muscle can be retracted far enough cranially, a plate may be applied to the lateral aspect of the ulna, without the additional lateral exposure between the ulnaris lateralis muscle and the lateral digital extensor muscle.

References

1. Adams, O. R.: Lameness in Horses. 3rd ed., Philadelphia, Lea and Febiger, 1974, pp. 167–168.
2. Fessler, J. F., and Amstutz, H. E. *In* Oehme, F. W., and Prier, J. E. (eds.): Large Animal Surgery. Baltimore, the Williams & Wilkins Company, 1974, pp. 312–314.
3. Fretz, P. B.: Fractured Ulna in the Horse. Can. Vet. J. *14* (1973):50–53.
4. Johnson, J. H. and Butler, H. C.: The Tension Band Principle in Fixation of an Equine Ulna Fracture. Vet. Med. Small Anim. Clin. *66* (1971):552–556.
5. Milne, D. W., Turner, A. S. and Gabel, A. A.: Surgical Approaches to Certain Long Bones of the Horse for Application of Tension Band Plates. J.A.V.M.A. *168*, (1976):48–52.
6. Monin, T.: Repair of Physeal Fractures of the Tuber Olecranon in the Horse, Using a Tension Band Method. J.A.V.M.A. *172*, 287–290, Feb. 1, 1978.
7. Scott, E. A.: "Tension-Band Fixation of Equine Ulna Fractures Using Semi-Tubular Plates." *In* Proceedings, 21st Annual Meeting, American Association Equine Practitioners, 1975. (1976):167–168.
8. Turner, A. S., Milne, D. W., and Gabel, A. A.: Use of the Dynamic Compression Plate for Treatment of Equine Longbone Fractures. J.A.V.M.A. *168*, (1976):309–315.

part eight

Approaches to the Radius

MEDIAL APPROACH TO THE DIAPHYSIS AND METAPHYSES OF THE RADIUS

INDICATION

1. Surgical repair of fractures of the radius.[1–7]

POSITIONING OF PATIENT

The horse is positioned in right or left lateral recumbency with the affected limb down.

DESCRIPTION OF PROCEDURE

A. *Topographical View.* A curvilinear incision approximately 30 cm. long is made through the skin on the medial aspect of the radius, from the medial tuberosity of the distal end of the radius to the point of attachment of the long medial ligament of the elbow. From the position of this eminence, the incision is continued cranioproximally along the ventral border of the caudal superficial pectoral muscle, for a distance of approximately 8 cm. The apex of the skin incision is directed caudally over the medial aspect of the flexor carpi radialis muscle, passing approximately 2 cm. from the chestnut. The base of the skin incision lies cranially over the cranial-medial aspect of the radius. This skin incision is made carefully, so as not to cut through the cephalic vein where it crosses the medial aspect of the radius between the chestnut and medial tuberosity of the distal end of the radius.

B. *Surgeon's View.* The skin is reflected from the apex of the incision toward the cranial-medial aspect of the radius. The superficial fascia contains the cephalic and accessory cephalic veins and the cutaneous branches of the musculocutaneous nerve. These structures should be left with the fascia when the skin is reflected. If the more proximal aspect of the radius needs to be exposed for the placement of a plate close to the elbow, the skin incision is extended caudally and proximally from the position for the attachment of the long medial ligament of the elbow, along the remaining border of the caudal superficial pectoral muscle. The subcutaneous incision is made along the border of the caudal superficial pectoral muscle, then extends down the cranial-medial aspect of the radius (cranial to the cephalic vein) to the medial tuberosity of the distal end of the radius.

MEDIAL APPROACH TO THE DIAPHYSIS AND METAPHYSES OF THE RADIUS

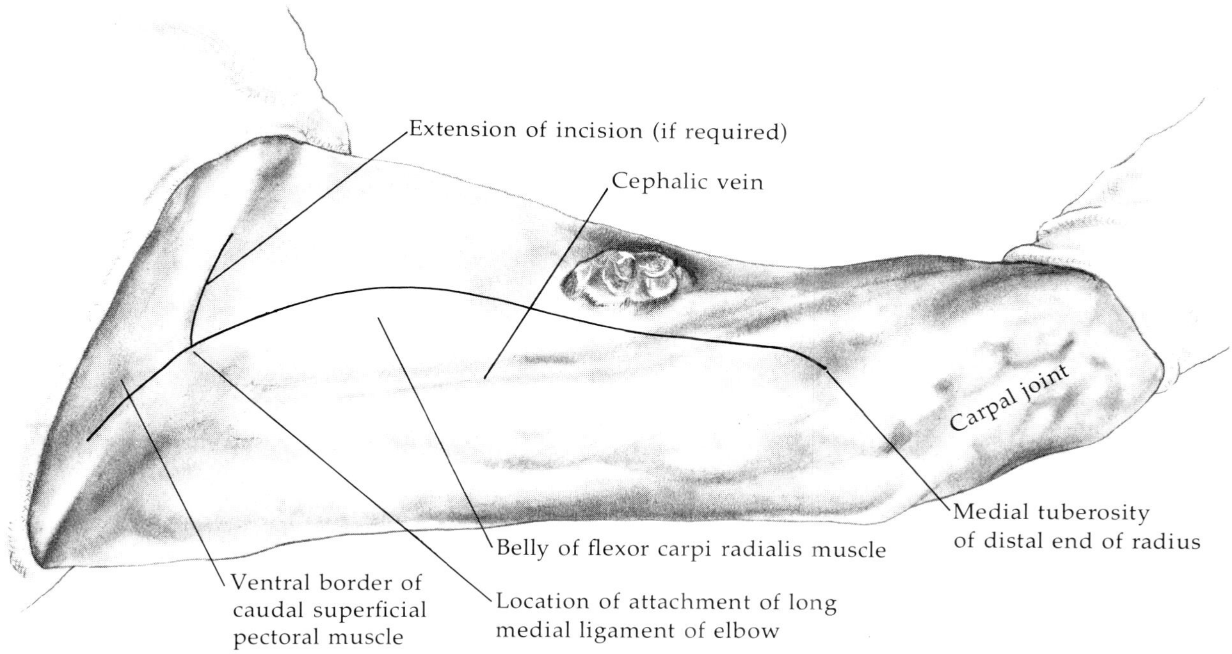

A

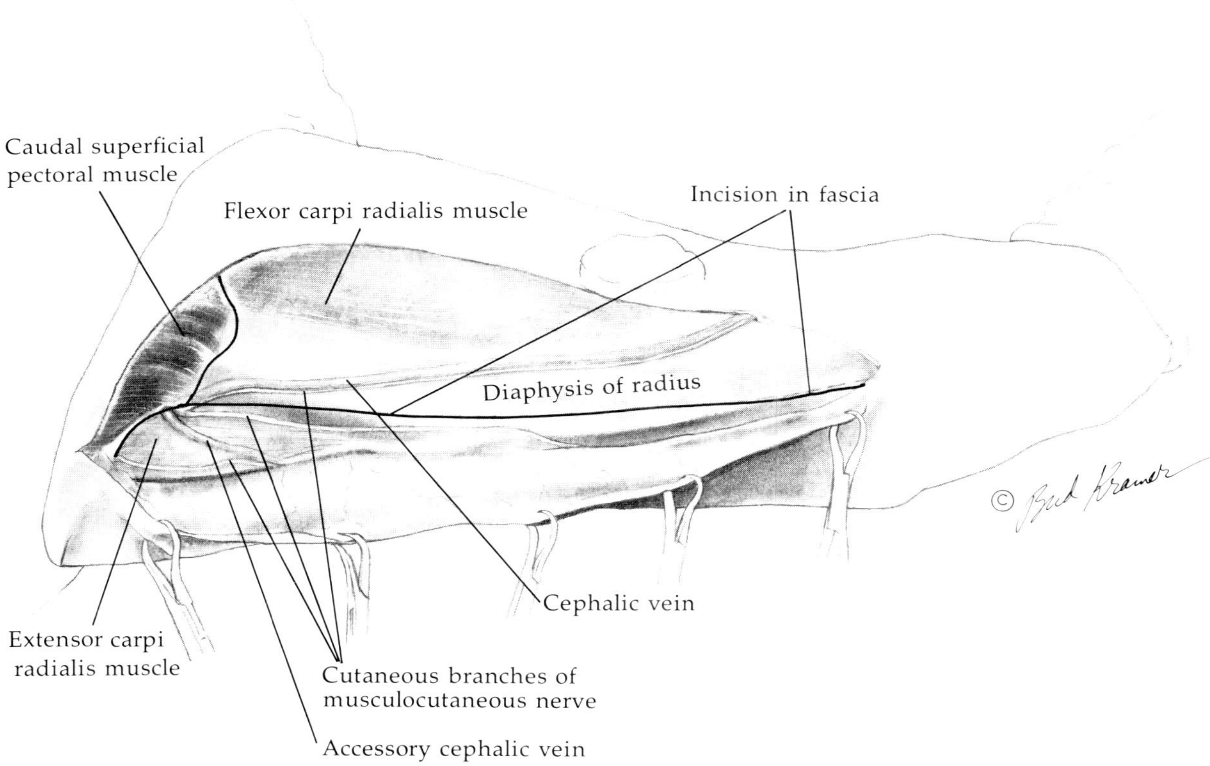

B

C. *Surgeon's View.* The cephalic vein and one of the cutaneous branches of the musculocutaneous nerve are reflected caudally along with half of the incised superficial fascia. The accessory cephalic vein and the other cutaneous branches of the musculocutaneous nerve are reflected cranially along with the other half of the incised superficial fascia. The caudal superficial pectoral muscle is reflected proximally to expose the proximal end of the radius, the long medial collateral ligament of the elbow, the attachment of the brachialis muscle, the median nerve, the brachial artery, and the satellite veins caudal to the long medial ligament of the elbow. To apply a plate to the most proximal part of the radius, the median nerve, brachial artery, and satellite veins must be reflected caudally, and the long medial ligament cranially, with the plate placed under the vein, artery, and nerve. To place a plate on the cranial-medial aspect of the radius, the extensor carpi radialis muscle must be reflected away from the radius.*

CLOSURE

The subcutaneous fascia is closed using an interrupted or continuous suture pattern. The skin is closed using an interrupted pattern with the incised edges in firm apposition.

COMMENTS

This approach will give access to the medial, cranial and cranial-medial aspect of the radius. Problems may arise when double plating is anticipated (as is usually the case) and a plate is placed under the distal aspect of the extensor carpi radialis muscle. Postoperative stiffness of the carpi may occur as a result of the implant impinging on the tendon of this muscle. For this reason, the lateral approach to the cranial-lateral aspect (the tension side) may be necessary along with the medial approach. This will allow the surgeon to place the plates lateral and medial to the tendon of the extensor carpi radialis muscle, reducing the chance of carpal stiffness. Simultaneous medial and lateral incisions will necessitate operating with the horse in dorsal recumbency with the leg extended upward.

References

1. Alexander, J. T., and Rooney R. J.: The Biomechanics, Surgery and Prognosis of Equine Fractures. *In* Proceedings, 18th Annual Meeting, American Association of Equine Practitioners, 1972. (1973): 219–235.
2. Dingwall, J. S., Duncan, D. B., and Horney, F. D.: Compression Plating in Large Animal Orthopedics. J.A.V.M.A. *158* (1971):1651–1657.
3. Fessler, J. F. and Amstutz, H. E. *In* Oehme, F. W., and Prier, J. E. (eds.): Large Animal Surgery. Baltimore, The Williams & Wilkins Company, 1974, pp. 309–312.
4. Gertson, K. E., and Brinker, W. O.: Fracture Repair in Ponies Using Bone Plates. J.A.V.M.A., *154* (1969):900–905.
5. Gertson, K. E., Monfort, J. N., and Tillotson, P. J.: Fracture Repair in Large Animals. Vet. Med. Small Anim. Clin. *68* (1973):782–790.
6. Milne, D. W., Turner, A. S., and Gabel, A. A.: Surgical Approaches to Certain Long Bones of the Horse for Application of Tension Band Plates. J.A.V.M.A. *168* (1976):48–52.
7. Turner, A. S., Milne, D. W., and Gabel, A. A.: The Dynamic Compression Plate in Equine Long Bone Fractures. J.A.V.M.A. *168* (1976):309–315.

*See Comments.

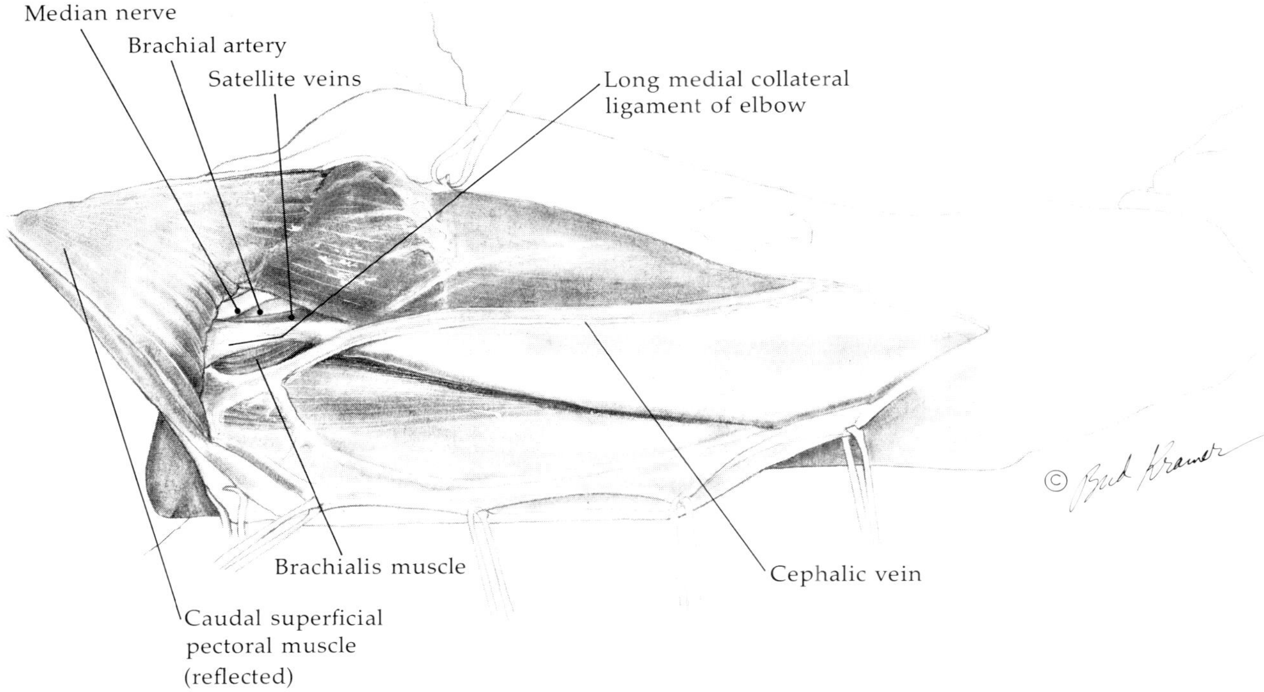
Median nerve
Brachial artery
Satellite veins
Long medial collateral ligament of elbow
Brachialis muscle
Cephalic vein
Caudal superficial pectoral muscle (reflected)
© Bud Kramer

C

LATERAL APPROACH TO THE DIAPHYSIS AND METAPHYSES OF THE RADIUS

INDICATION

1. Open reduction and fixation of fractures of the radius.[1-7]

POSITIONING OF PATIENT

The patient is positioned with the affected limb uppermost.

DESCRIPTION OF PROCEDURE

A. *Topographical View.* A skin incision approximately 30 cm. long is made, extending from the lateral condyle of the distal humerus to just proximal to the cranial aspect of the lateral tuberosity for the attachment of the collateral ligament of the carpal joint. The skin is reflected cranially and caudally from the subcutaneous fascia to expose the fascial plane between the common digital extensor muscle and the extensor carpi radialis muscle.

B. *Diagrammatic View.* The subcutaneous fascia and the intermuscular septum between the common digital extensor and the extensor carpi radialis muscles are incised. This incision extends from just distal to the tuberosity for the attachment of the collateral ligament of the elbow joint to just proximal to the lateral tuberosity for the attachment of the collateral ligament of the carpal joint.

LATERAL APPROACH TO THE DIAPHYSIS AND METAPHYSES OF THE RADIUS

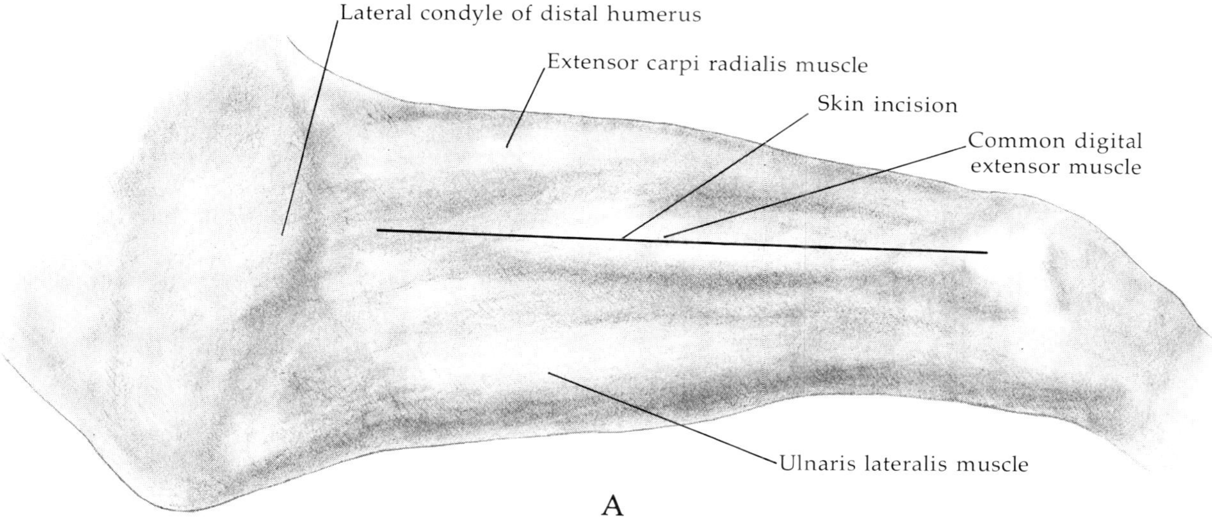

A

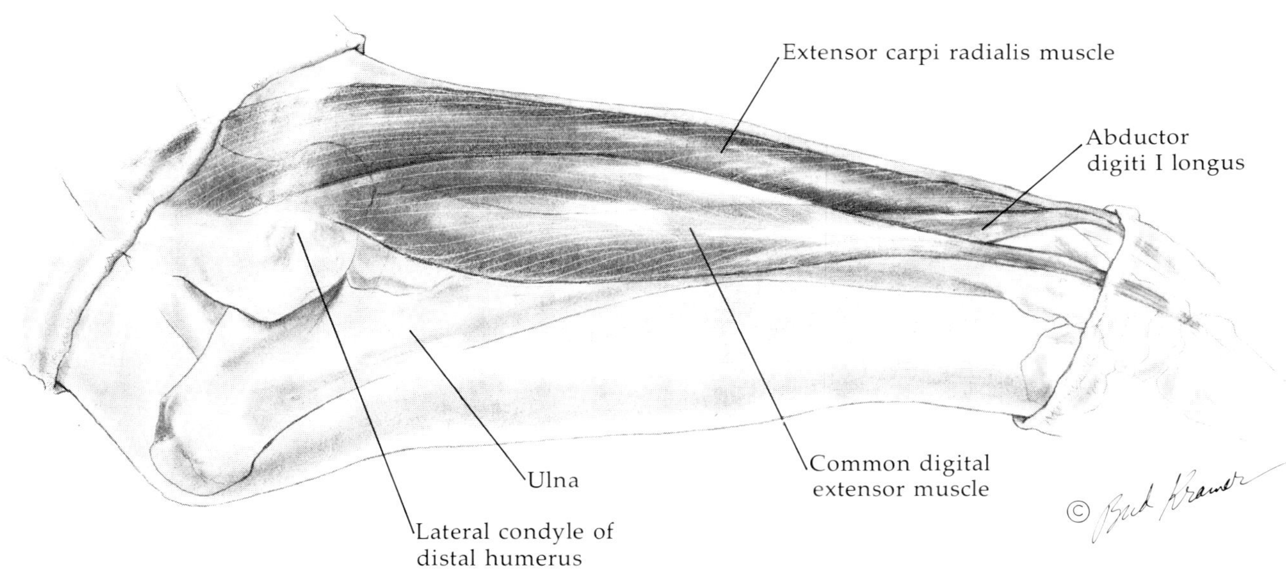

B

C. Surgeon's View. Once the intermuscular septum between the common digital extensor and extensor carpi radialis muscles is incised, blunt finger dissection is used to separate the muscle bellies for the length of the incision. To expose the cranial-lateral aspect of the radius, the extensor carpi radialis muscle is retracted cranially and the common digital extensor muscle caudally. The muscle belly of the abductor digiti I longus (extensor carpi obliquus) is closely adhered to the lateral aspect of the distal radius. This is visible once the common digital extensor is retracted caudally. Branches of the anastomotic loop of the transverse cubital and cranial interosseous artery and vein descend on the cranial surface of the radius under cover of the common digital extensor muscle, and supply branches to the extensor carpi radialis muscle at the junction of the middle and proximal thirds of the radius. These vessels should be identified and preserved.

CLOSURE

The intermuscular fascial septum and subcutaneous fascia are closed using an interrupted or continuous suture pattern. The skin is closed using a simple interrupted suture pattern with the incised edges in firm apposition.

COMMENTS

This approach is used to place a bone plate on the cranial-lateral aspect (tension band side) of the radius.[6] It can be used in conjunction with a cranial-medial approach when more than one bone plate is required to establish rigid internal fixation of radial fractures.

Simultaneous medial and lateral incisions will necessitate operating with the horse in dorsal recumbency, with the leg extended upward.

References

1. Alexander, J. T., and Rooney, R. J.: The Biomechanics, Surgery and Prognosis of Equine Fractures. *In* Proceedings, 18th Annual Meeting, American Association Equine Practitioners, 1972. (1973):219–235.
2. Dingwall, J. S., Duncan, D. B., and Horney, F. D.: Compression Plating in Large Animal Orthopedics. J.A.V.M.A. *158* (1971):1651–1657.
3. Fessler, J. F. and Amstutz, H. E. *In* Oehme, F. W., and Prier, J. E. (eds.): Large Animal Surgery. Baltimore, The Williams & Wilkins Company, 1974. 309–312.
4. Gertson, K. E., and Brinker, W. O.: Fracture Repair in Ponies Using Bone Plates. J.A.V.M.A. *154* (1969):900–905.
5. Gertson, K. E., Monfort, J. N., and Tillotson, P. J.: Fracture Repair in Large Animals. Vet. Med. Small Anim. Clin. *68* (1973):782–790.
6. Milne, D. W., Turner, A. S., and Gabel, A. A.: Surgical Approaches to Certain Long Bones of the Horse for Application of Tension Band Plates. J.A.V.M.A. *168* (1976):48–52.
7. Turner, A. S., Milne, D. W., and Gabel, A. A.: The Dynamic Compression Plate in Equine Long Bone Fractures. J.A.V.M.A. *168* (1976):309–315.

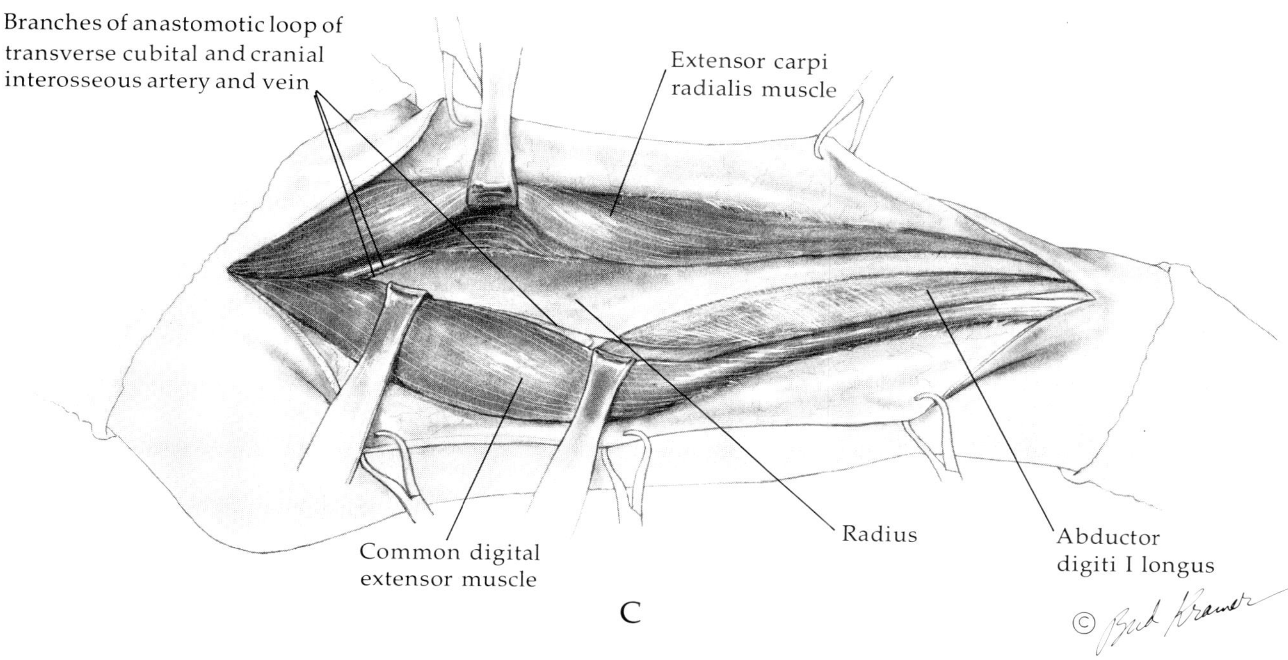
Branches of anastomotic loop of transverse cubital and cranial interosseous artery and vein
Extensor carpi radialis muscle
Common digital extensor muscle
Radius
Abductor digiti I longus
© Bud Kramer

C

part nine

Approach to the Humerus

LATERAL APPROACH TO THE DIAPHYSIS AND METAPHYSES OF THE HUMERUS

INDICATION

1. Open reduction and fixation of fractures of the humerus in foals.[1-3]

POSITIONING OF THE PATIENT

The foal is positioned in lateral recumbency with the affected leg uppermost.

DESCRIPTION OF PROCEDURE

A. *Topographical View.* An incision approximately 24 cm. long is made from the greater tubercle of the humerus to the lateral epicondyle of the humerus. The incision lies cranial to the cranial border of the triceps brachii muscle. The subcutaneous fascia is incised along the same line as the skin incision.

B. *Surgeon's View.* To expose the proximal third of the humerus, a plane of dissection is commenced under the caudal border of the brachiocephalicus muscle. Reflection of the brachiocephalicus muscle cranially will reveal the anterior border of the brachialis muscle. A plane of dissection is established along its anterior border and the muscle is retracted caudally; the brachiocephalicus is retracted cranially. Because of the close apposition of the brachialis muscle to the musculospiral groove of the humerus, exposure of the middle third of the humerus is difficult.

LATERAL APPROACH TO THE DIAPHYSIS AND METAPHYSES OF THE HUMERUS

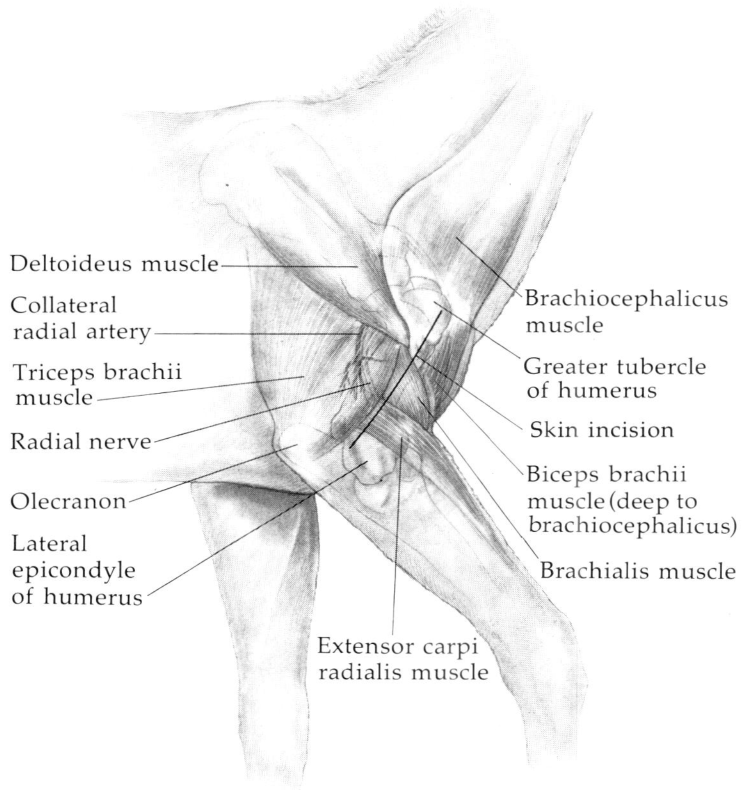

A

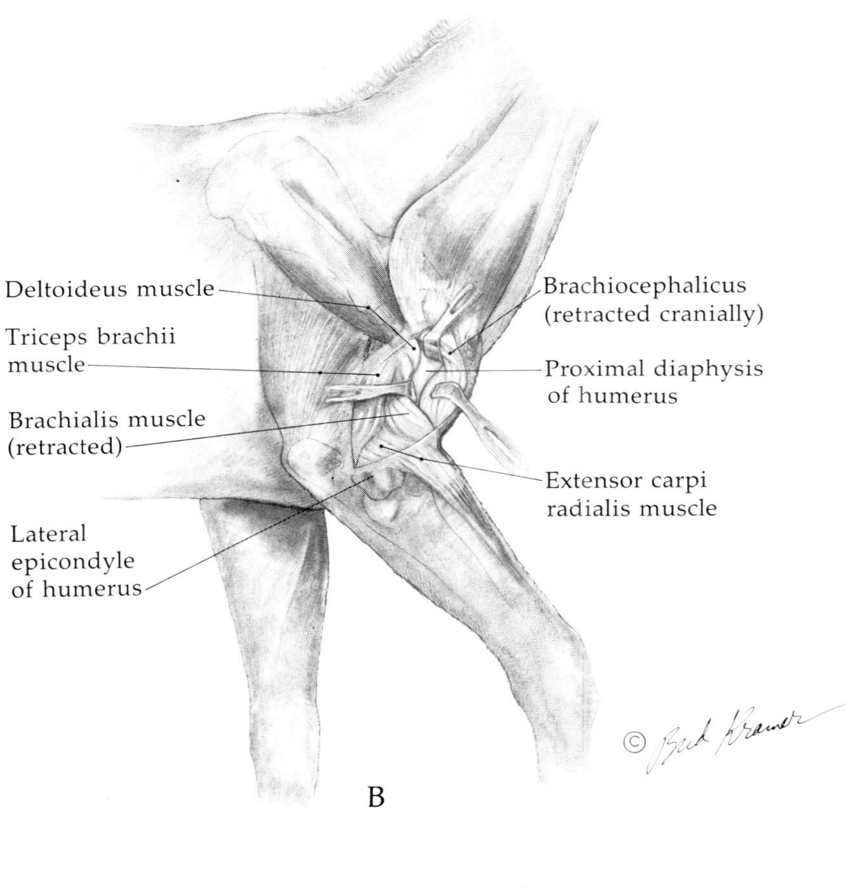

B

C. Surgeon's View. To expose the distal third of the humerus, the brachialis muscle is retracted cranially and the triceps brachii is retracted caudally. In addition, the extensor carpi radialis muscle is retracted caudoventrally.

D and E. Schematic View. When exposing the distal third of the humerus, the radial nerve and collateral radial artery should be identified and preserved. These structures run craniodistally and are in close apposition to the bone in the musculospiral groove of the humerus deep to the triceps brachii and the head of the extensor carpi radialis muscles.

CLOSURE

The caudal border of the brachiocephalicus muscle is sutured to the surrounding fascia using a continuous or interrupted pattern. The subcutaneous fascia is closed using a continuous suture pattern. The skin is closed using an interrupted suture pattern with the incised edges in firm apposition.

COMMENTS

The humerus of the horse is very short and curved. This anatomical feature, in addition to the middle third being covered by the brachialis muscle, makes this a difficult bone for use of conventional internal fixation devices. Because of the large muscle mass which immobilizes the humerus of the horse, many fractures of the mid-shaft of the humerus in young, immature horses (< 180 kg) will heal without internal or external coaptations.

References

1. Alexander, J. T., and Rooney, J. R.: The Biomechanics, Surgery and Prognosis of Equine Fractures. *In* Proceedings, 18th Annual Meeting, American Association of Equine Practitioners, 1972. (1973):219–235.
2. Fessler, J. F., and Amstutz, H. E. *In* Oehme, F. W., and Prier, J. E. (eds.): Large Animal Surgery. Baltimore, the Williams & Wilkins Company, 1974, pp. 314–316.
3. Vaughan, L. C.: Limb Injuries in Foals. Equine Vet. J. *1*(3) (1968):4–8.

LATERAL APPROACH TO THE DIAPHYSIS AND METAPHYSES OF THE HUMERUS

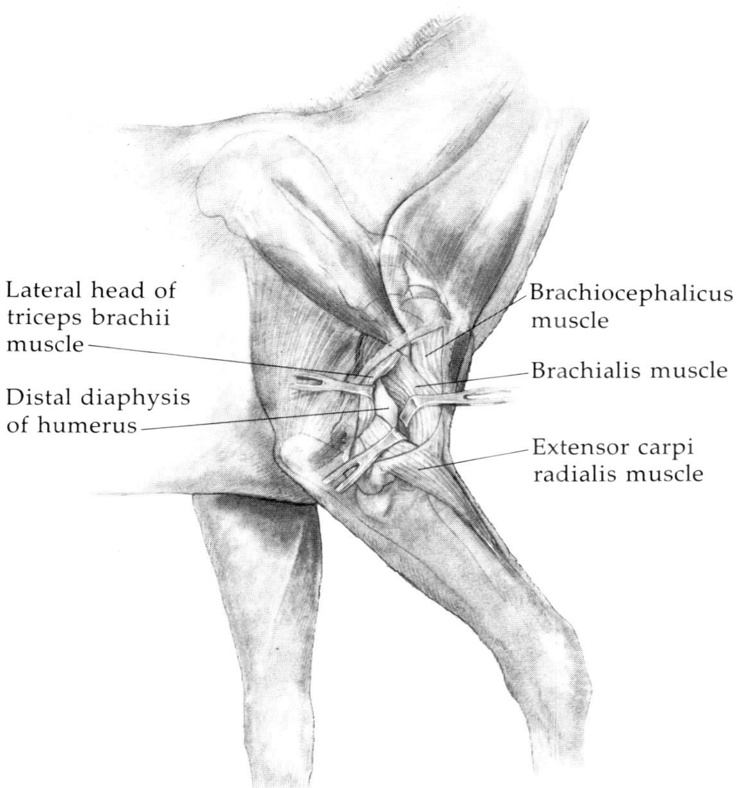

C

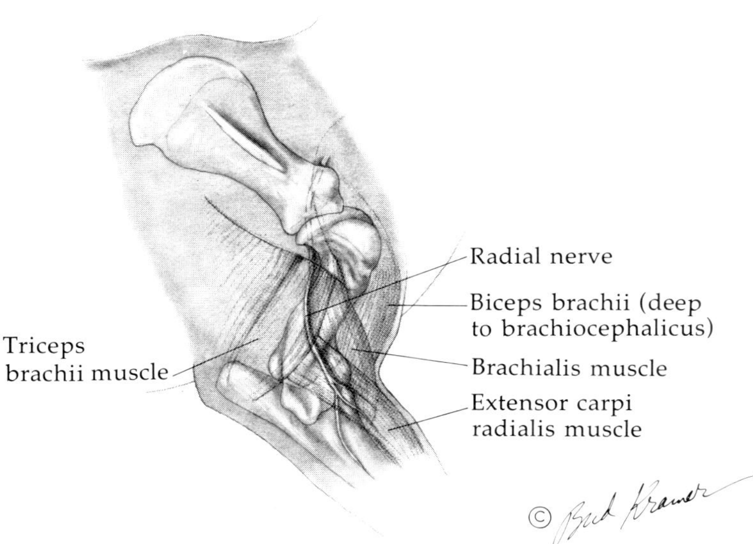

D

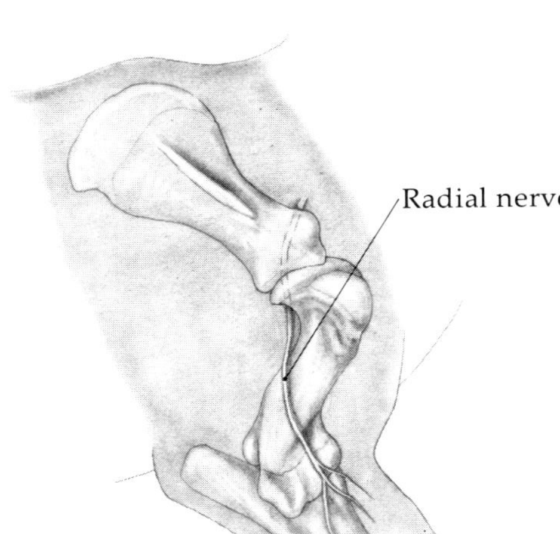

E

part ten

Approach to the Tuber Scapulae

LATERAL APPROACH TO THE TUBER SCAPULAE OF THE GLENOID FOSSA

INDICATIONS

1. Open reduction and fixation of fractures of the tuber scapulae.[1]
2. Surgical excision of the tuber scapulae.[1]

POSITIONING OF PATIENT

The horse is positioned in lateral recumbency with the affected limb uppermost.

DESCRIPTION OF PROCEDURE

A. *Topographical View.* An incision approximately 20 cm. long is made, extending from the junction of the middle and distal thirds of the spine of the scapula to the greater tubercle of the humerus. The incision lies just cranial to the spine of the scapula running parallel to the caudal-lateral border of the supraspinatus muscle.

LATERAL APPROACH TO THE TUBER SCAPULAE OF THE GLENOID FOSSA

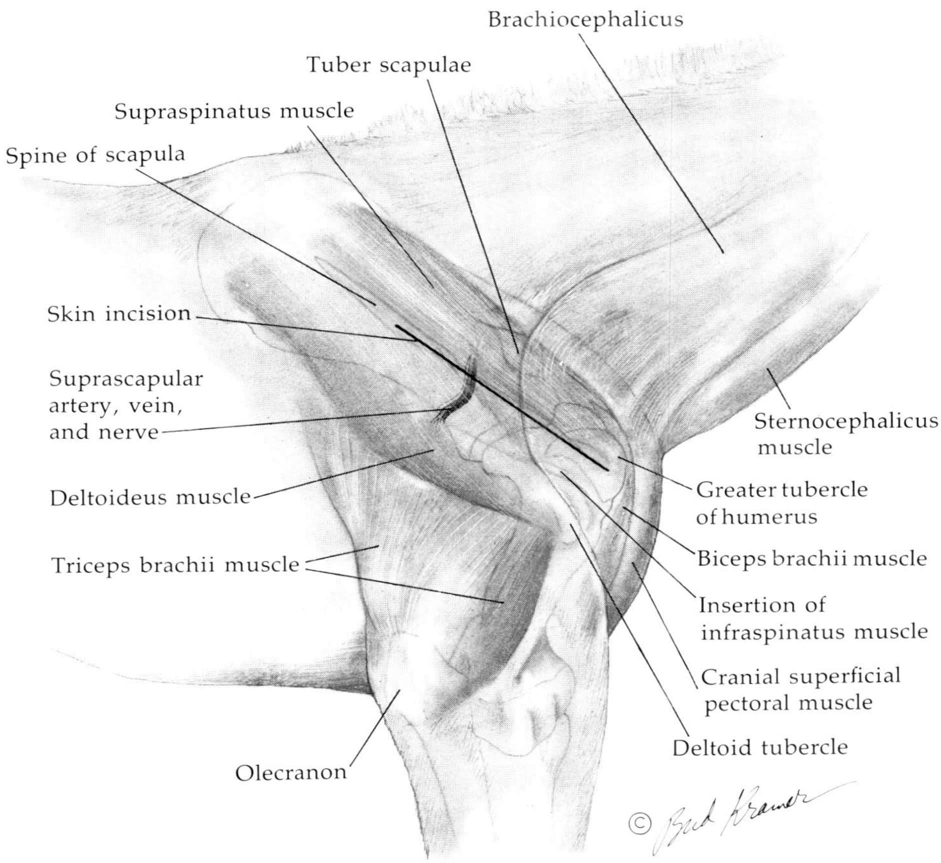

A

LATERAL APPROACH TO THE TUBER SCAPULAE OF THE GLENOID FOSSA

B and C. Surgeon's View. The subcutaneous fascia, the deep fascia, and the superficial aponeurosis of the supraspinatus muscle are incised along the same line as the skin incision. The caudal border of the brachiocephalicus muscle is reflected cranially. The supraspinatus muscle is closely adhered to the lateral aspect of the scapula in the supraspinous fossa. To expose the attachment of the tendon of the biceps brachii on the tuber scapulae, the caudal border of the supraspinatus muscle is subperiosteally elevated and reflected cranially, the infraspinatus is reflected caudodistally and the deltoideus caudally. Care must be taken to preserve the suprascapular nerve, artery, and vein. These structures turn around the distal fourth of the cranial border of the scapula, giving branches to the supraspinatus muscle and continuing caudally to innervate the infraspinatus muscle.

CLOSURE

The superficial aponeurosis of the supraspinatus muscle is closed, using an interrupted or continuous suture pattern. The deep fascia of the shoulder and the caudal edge of the brachiocephalicus muscle are reattached, using an interrupted or continuous suture pattern. The subcutaneous fascia is closed, using a continuous suture pattern. The skin is closed using an interrupted pattern. Tension sutures are used in addition because of excessive motion occurring at the skin incision as the shoulder joint is moved. This helps prevent postoperative wound dehiscence.

COMMENTS

Fractures of the tuber scapulae are not uncommon and occur from overextension of the tendon of the biceps brachii muscle. Internal fixation of the tuber scapulae with adequate rigid immobilization is extremely difficult to obtain because of the mechanical forces of the biceps brachii muscle which distracts it. Also, the complicated shape of the distal scapula makes internal fixation difficult. Because of repeated failures with internal fixation, surgical excision has been performed.[1] This requires incising the tendon of the biceps brachii muscle from its attachment to the tuber scapulae.

Reference

1. Lietch, M. A.: A Review of Treatment of Tuber Scapulae Fractures in the Horse. J. Equine Med. Surg. *1* (6): (1977):234–240.

LATERAL APPROACH TO THE TUBER SCAPULAE OF THE GLENOID FOSSA

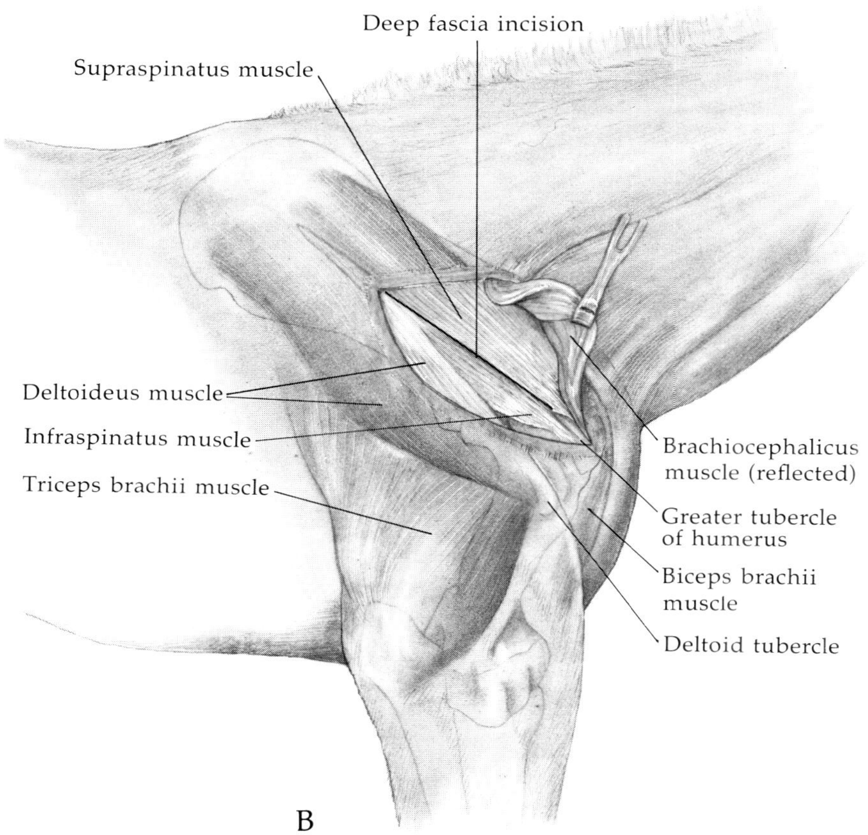

B

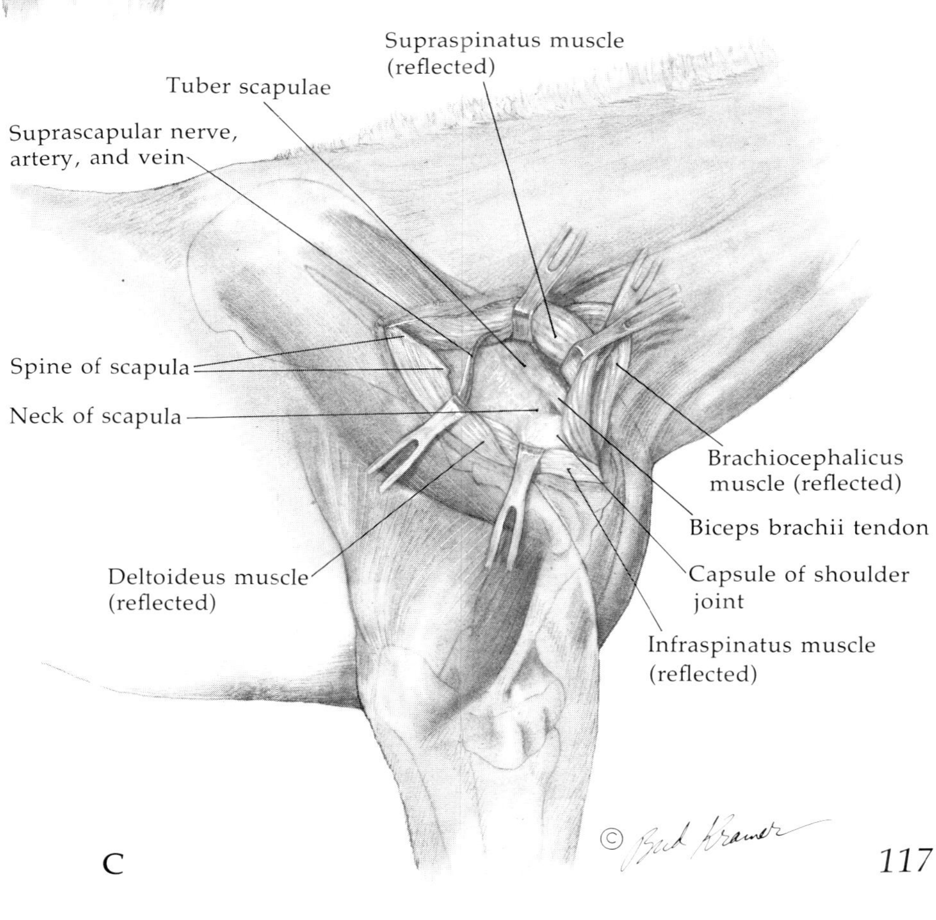

C

section three

THE PELVIC LIMB

part one

Approaches to the Third and Fourth Metatarsal Bones

LATERAL APPROACH TO THE THIRD METATARSUS

INDICATION

1. Open reduction and internal fixation of fractures of the third metatarsus.

POSITIONING OF PATIENT

The patient is placed with the affected limb uppermost.

DESCRIPTION OF PROCEDURE

A. *Topographical View.* A curvilinear incision approximately 30 cm. long is made through the skin on the lateral aspect of Mt III, from the lateral prominence of the condyle of Mt III to the proximal-cranial aspect of Mt IV.

B. *Surgeon's View.* The apex of the skin incision is directed caudally over the lateral aspect of the interosseous (suspensory) ligament and the deep digital flexor tendon; the base of the incision lies cranially over the cranial-lateral aspect of the metatarsus. The skin incision is made carefully, so as not to extend through the lateral dorsal metatarsal artery and nerve where they cross obliquely over the proximal-lateral aspect of the metatarsus. The skin is reflected cranially from the apex toward the cranial-lateral aspect of the Mt III. A straight incision is made through the superficial fascia over the third metatarsal shaft, extending from the lateral prominence of the condyle of Mt III to the proximal-cranial aspect of Mt IV. To facilitate placement of the plate at the proximal end of the Mt III, the tendon of the lateral digital extensor muscle is reflected cranially, the dorsal metatarsal artery and nerve are reflected caudally, and the distal extensor retinaculum is reflected proximally.

CLOSURE

The subcutaneous fascia is closed with an interrupted or continuous suture pattern. The skin should be closed with an interrupted suture pattern with the incised edges in firm apposition.

COMMENTS

The lateral approach is used for fractures of Mt III because the tension band side lies on the cranial-lateral aspect of this bone.[6]

References

1. Alexander, J. T., and Rooney, R. J.: The Biomechanics, Surgery and Prognosis of Equine Fractures. *In* Proceedings, 18th Annual Meeting, American Association. Equine Practitioners, 1972. (1973): 219–235.
2. Dingwall, J. S., Duncan, D. B., and Horney, F. D.: Compression Plating in Large Animal Orthopedics. J.A.V.M.A. *158*(1971):1651–1657.
3. Fessler, J. F., and Amstutz, H. E.: *In* Oehme, F. W., and Prier, J. E. (eds.): Large Animal Surgery, Baltimore, The Williams & Wilkins Company, 1974 pp. 309–312.
4. Gertson, K. E., and Brinker, W. O.: Fracture Repair in Ponies Using Bone Plates. J.A.V.M.A. *154*(1969):900–905.
5. Gertson, K. E., Monfort, J. N., and Tillotson, P. J.: Fracture Repair in Large Animals. Vet. Med. Small Anim. Clin. *68*(1973):782–790.
6. Milne, D. W., Turner, A. S., and Gabel, A. A. Surgical Approaches to Certain Long Bones of the Horse for Application of Tension Band Plates. J.A.V.M.A. *168*(1976):48–52.
7. Turner, A. S., Milne, D. W., and Gabel, A. A.: The Dynamic Compression Plate in Equine Long Bone Fractures. J.A.V.M.A. *168*(1976):309–315.

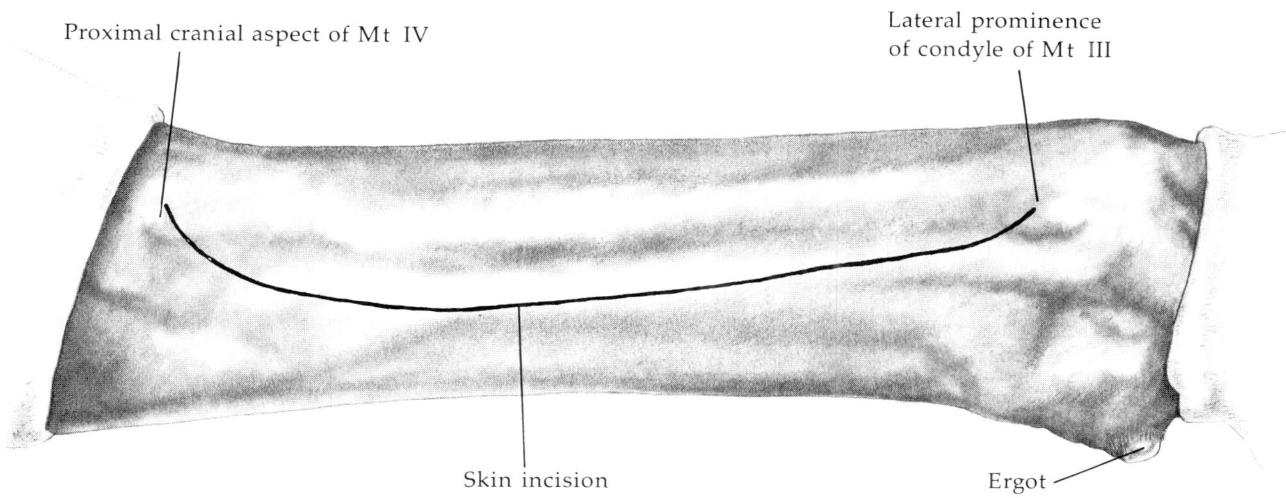

Proximal cranial aspect of Mt IV
Lateral prominence of condyle of Mt III
Skin incision
Ergot

A

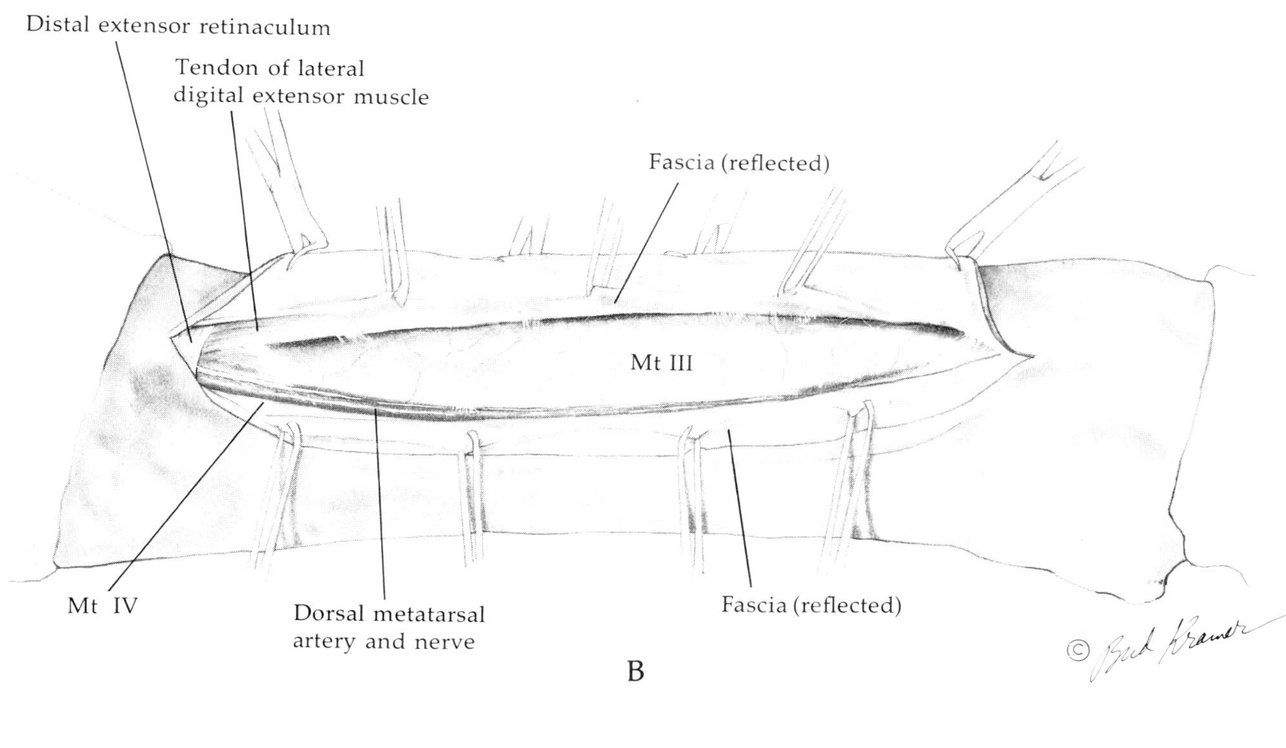

Distal extensor retinaculum
Tendon of lateral digital extensor muscle
Fascia (reflected)
Mt III
Mt IV
Dorsal metatarsal artery and nerve
Fascia (reflected)

B

LATERAL APPROACH TO THE FOURTH METATARSUS (LATERAL SPLINT BONE)

INDICATIONS

1. Surgical excision of the distal fragment of fractures of Mt IV.[1–3, 5]
2. Surgical excision of bone sequestra involving Mt IV.[1, 4]

POSITIONING OF PATIENT

The horse is positioned in left or right lateral recumbency with the affected limb uppermost.

DESCRIPTION OF PROCEDURE

A. Topographical View. A variable length skin incision is made directly over the lateral aspect of Mt IV extending from approximately 1 cm. distal to the distal extremity of this bone to approximately 2 cm. proximal to the proposed site of amputation.

B. Surgeon's View. The subcutaneous fascia is incised along the same line as the skin incision, extending to, but not through, the periosteum covering Mt IV. Once the skin and subcutaneous fascia are incised and retracted, Mt IV should be immediately visible.

LATERAL APPROACH TO THE FOURTH METATARSUS (LATERAL SPLINT BONE)

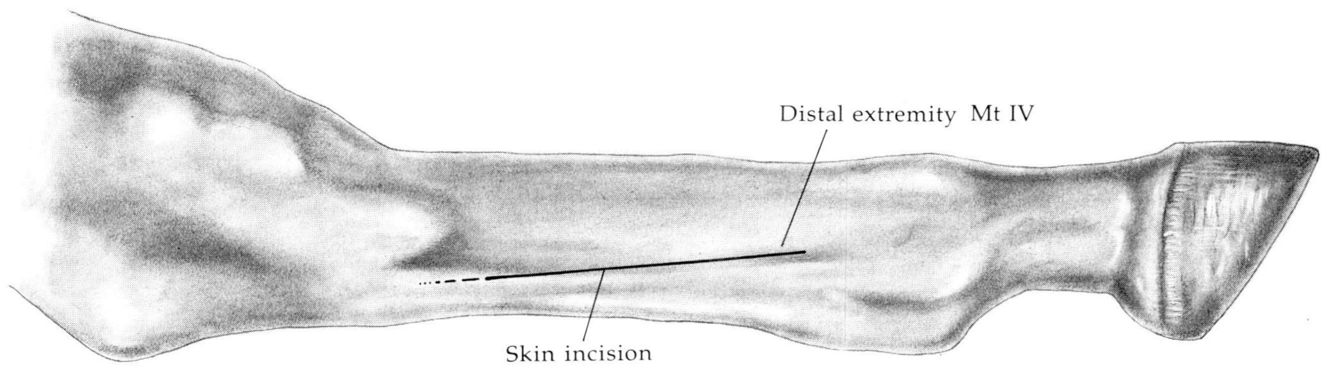

A

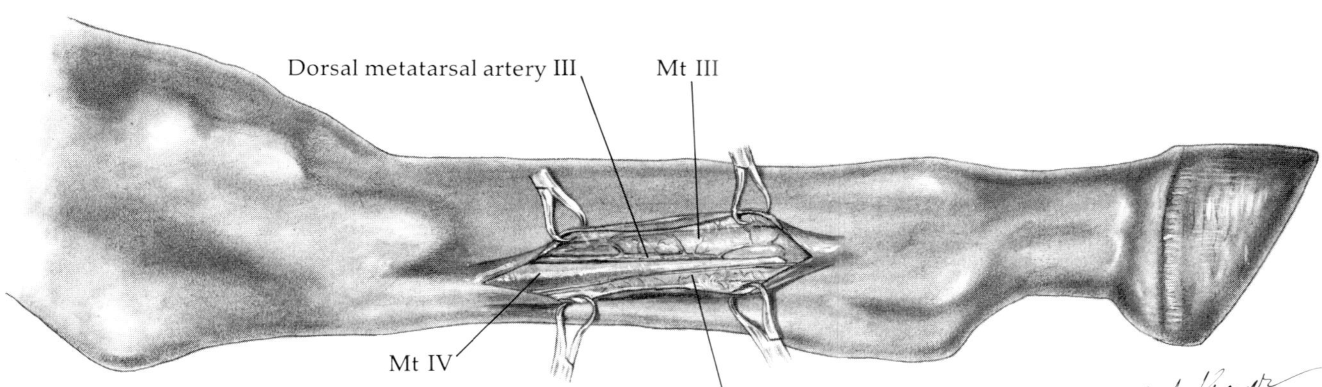

B

C. *Diagrammatic View of Tendons and Ligaments in Relationship to Bones.* When removing the distal portion of Mt IV, care must be taken not to incise through the interosseous ligament lying caudal-medial to Mt IV. When dissecting the most distal portion of the fourth metatarsus free, the small interosseous tendon is incised or retracted as it passes over the distal extremity of Mt IV.

D. *Diagrammatic View of Vessels in Relationship to Tendons, Ligaments and Bones.* The large, dorsal metatarsal artery III (great metatarsal artery) lies above and between Mt III and Mt IV in the interosseous space. It should be protected, and retracted cranially when Mt IV is amputated. The plantar metatarsal vein lies deep and medial to Mt IV, passing close to its distal extremity. Care should be taken to preserve this vein; it can usually be avoided if the surgeon does not dissect too far medially to Mt IV when removing the distal fragment. The lateral plantar vein is far enough caudal to be out of the plane of dissection.

CLOSURE

An interrupted or continuous pattern is used to close the subcutaneous fascia. The skin should be closed with an interrupted pattern with the incised edges in firm apposition.

COMMENTS

When excising the distal fragment for Mt IV fractures, the surgeon may choose to dissect the bone out of its surrounding periosteum, and then suture it closed after removal of the distal fragment.[1] This procedure is time consuming and does not appear to be necessary. It is recommended that the periosteum be removed along with the distal fragment.

Removal of the distal fragment of Mt IV is difficult owing to the relationship of the large dorsal metatarsal artery III. The surgeon must be careful to preserve this artery when incising in the interosseous space to free the attachments of Mt IV from Mt III.

The approach to Mt IV is described because of the proximity of this large artery to the area of dissection. The approach to Mt II is essentially the same, without the encumbrance of this large vessel.

References

1. Adams, O. R.: Lameness in Horses. 3rd ed., Philadelphia, Lea and Febiger, 1974, pp. 210–213.
2. Jones, R. D., and Fessler, J. F.: Observations on Small Metacarpal and Metatarsal Fractures With or Without Associated Suspensory Desmitis in Standardbred Horses. Can. Vet. J. *18*(2)(1977):29–32.
3. Numans, S. R., and Wintzer, H. J.: Surgical Treatment of Splint Bone Fractures. Tierarz. Wchschr. *71*(11) (1961):205–210.
4. Rose, R. J.: Surgical Treatment of Osteomyelitis in the Metacarpal and Metatarsal Bones of the Horse. Vet. Rec. *102* (1978):498–500.
5. Wintzer, H. J.: Fractures of Equine Small Metacarpal or Metatarsal Bones. Tierarz. Wchschr. *73* (13) (1960):244.

LATERAL APPROACH TO THE FOURTH METATARSUS (LATERAL SPLINT BONE)

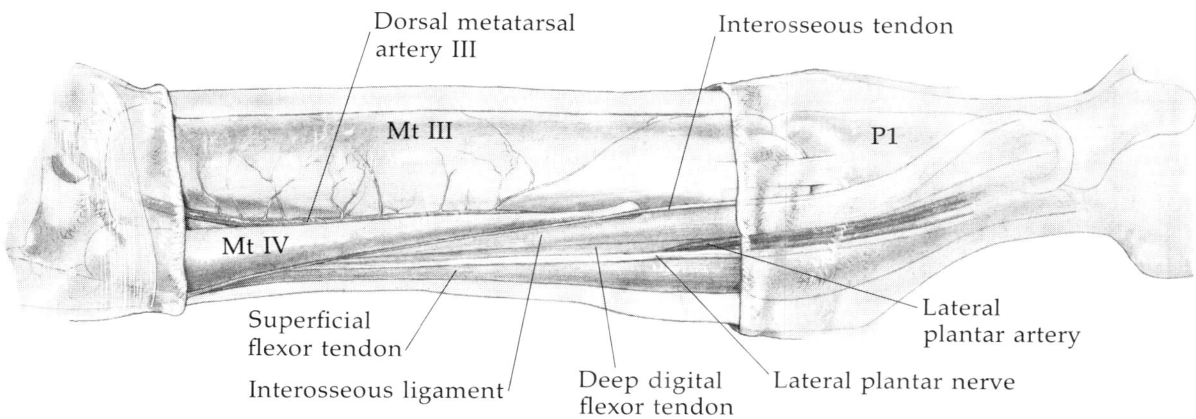

C

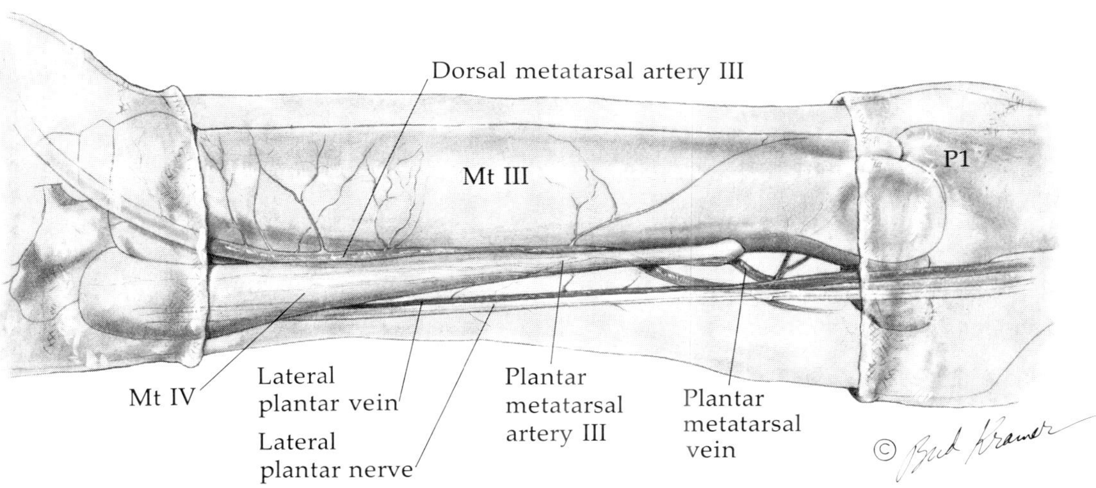

D

part two

Approaches to the Tarsus

CRANIOLATERAL APPROACH TO THE TIBIOTARSAL JOINT

INDICATIONS

1. Removal of chip fractures of the lateral and medial trochlea of the talus (tibiotarsal bone).[1–5]
2. Surgical curettage and removal of osteochondritic lesions and fragments from the lateral and medial trochlea of the talus and the middle sagittal ridge of the distal tibia.[1–5]
3. Removal of chip fractures of the lateral malleolus of the distal tibia.[1–5]

POSITIONING OF PATIENT

The patient is positioned with the affected limb uppermost.

DESCRIPTION OF PROCEDURE

A. *Topographical View.* An 8 cm. skin incision is made over the cranial-lateral aspect of the tibiotarsal joint, lateral to the tendon of the long digital extensor muscle. The incision extends from the level of the lateral malleolus of the tibia, to the level of the middle extensor retinaculum (annular ligament) and the lateral tendon of the fibularis (peroneus) tertius, which lies directly below the former.

B. *Diagrammatic View of Ligaments and Tendons in Relation to Bones.* The subcutaneous fascia and joint capsule are incised from the distal lateral malleolus of the tibia to the proximal border of the middle extensor retinaculum (annular ligament) and the lateral tendon of the fibularis (peroneus) tertius.

CRANIOLATERAL APPROACH TO THE TIBIOTARSAL JOINT

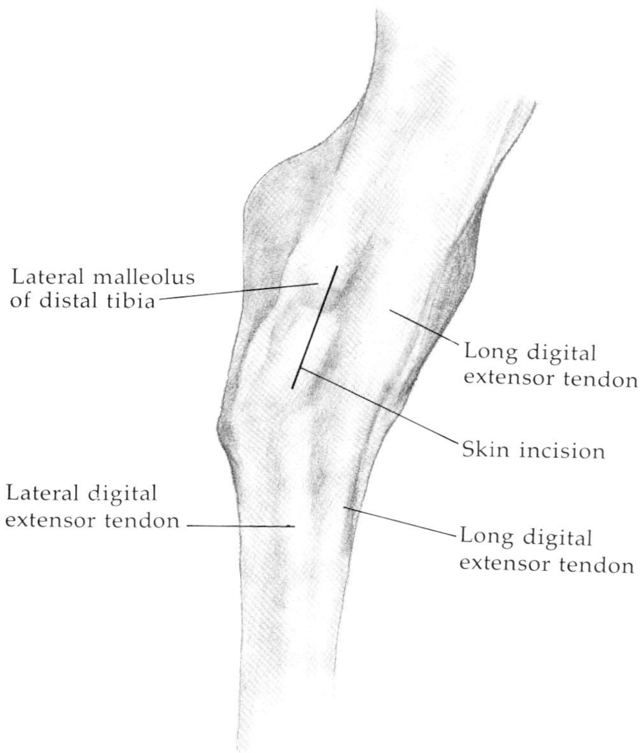

A

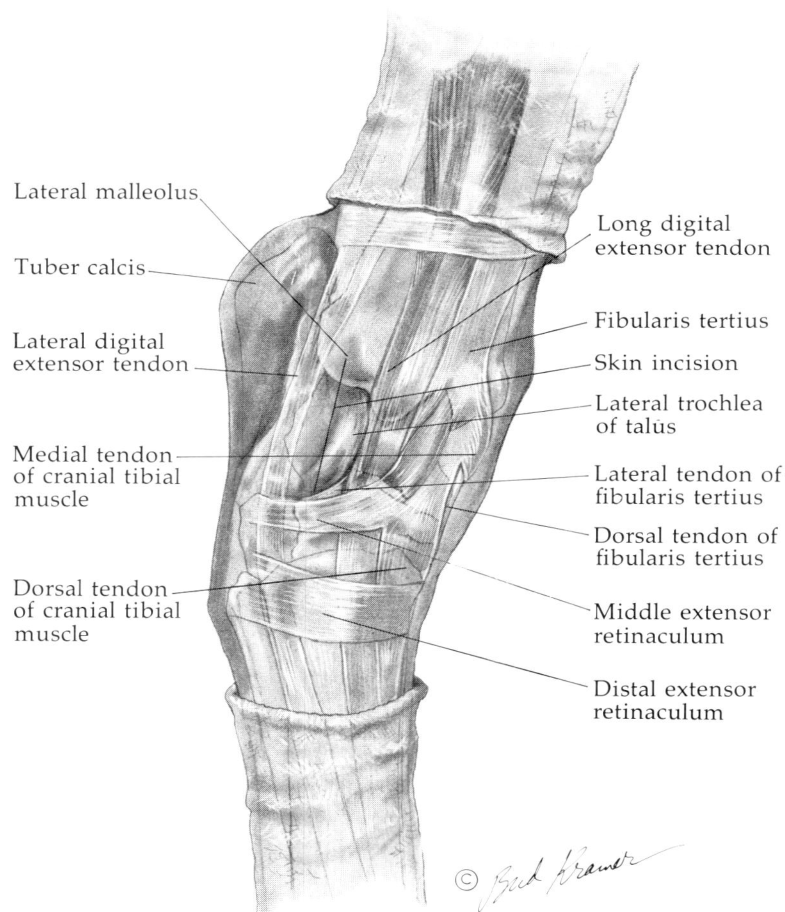

B

C. Surgeon's View. The cranial tibial vein passes along the lateral border of the long digital extensor tendon. The cranial tibial artery and deep fibular (peroneal) nerve pass behind the long digital extensor tendon. When making the incision in the skin, subcutaneous fascia, and joint capsule, and when retracting the edges of the incision, care should be taken to avoid injury to these structures.

D and E. Surgeon's View. The two margins of the joint capsule are retracted laterally and medially as the hock joint is flexed. Placing the tibiotarsal joint in hyperflexion will allow sufficient retraction of the margins of the incision to expose the lateral and medial trochlea of the talus.

CLOSURE

The joint capsule, subcutaneous tissues, and skin should be closed separately. The sutures in the joint capsule should not penetrate the synovial membrane; the synovial membrane of the joint capsule should not be allowed to evert between the opposed edges of the joint capsule as this reduces the rate and strength of healing.[4] Preplacement of the sutures in the joint capsule will allow a more accurate approximation of the cut edges of the joint capsule and achieve a tight seal (each suture is tied after all the sutures have been placed). An interrupted pattern is recommended for closure of the joint capsule; an interrupted or continuous pattern can be used to close the subcutaneous fascia. The skin should be closed with an interrupted pattern so that the edges are in firm apposition.

COMMENTS

The advantage of the cranial-lateral approach is good exposure of the articular surface of both the lateral and medial trochlea of the talus.

References

1. Birkeland, R., and Haakenstad, L. H.: Intracapsular Bony Fragments of the Distal Tibia of the Horse. J.A.V.M.A. *152*(1968):1526–1529.
2. Carter, E. I., Horney, F. D., and Pennock, P. W.: Distal Tibial Fractures in the Horse. Mod. Vet. Pract. (1972):41–42.
3. De Moor, A., Verschooten, F., Desmet, P., and Steenhaut, M.: Osteochondritis Dissecans of the Tibio-Tarsal Joint in the Horse. Equine Vet. J. *4*(1972):139–143.
4. International Symposium of Sutures in Wound Repair. London, England, Ethicon, U.S.A. July, 1972.
5. Schebitz, H., Dammrich, K., Waibl, H.: Intra-articular Fractures of the Hock Joint in Horses. Tierarztl. Wschr. *88*(1975):309–317.
6. Wheat, J. D. Fractures of the Trochlea of the Tibiotarsal Bone in the Horse. Proc. 100th Ann. Meet. A.V.M.A.:86–87, 1963.

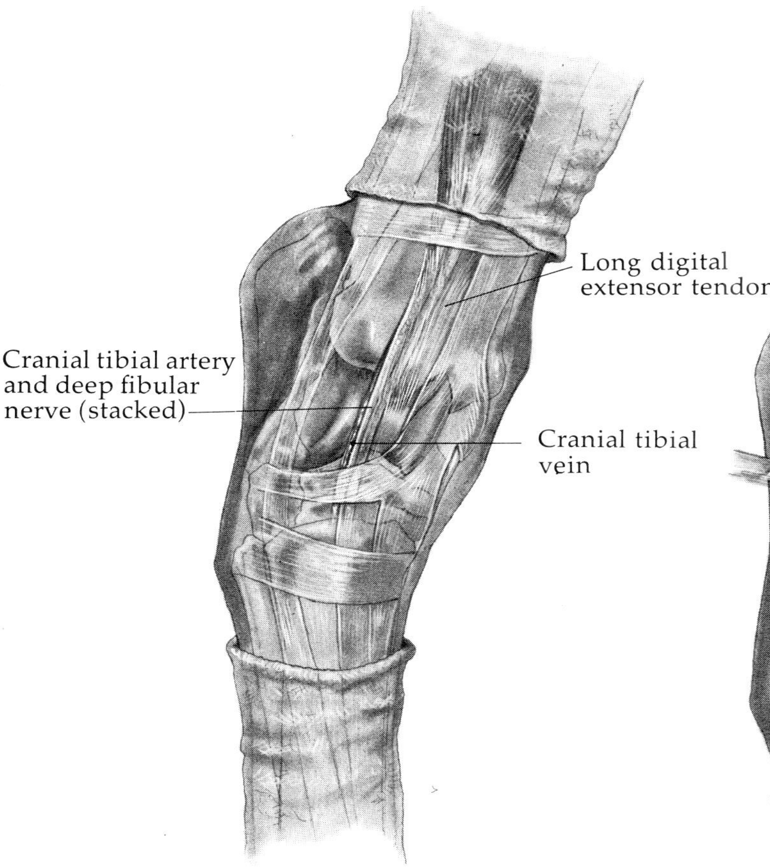

C

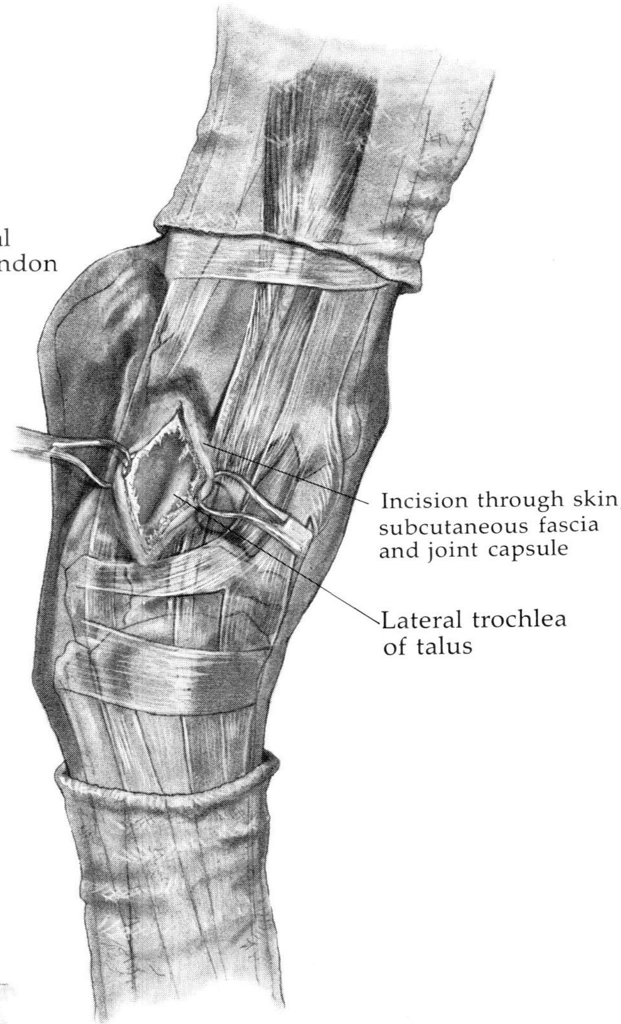

D

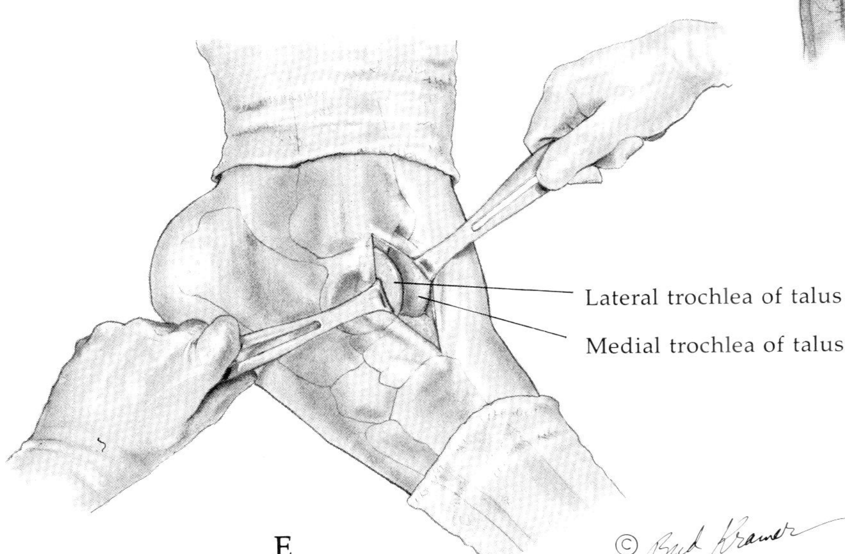

E

© Bud Kramer

CRANIOMEDIAL APPROACH TO TIBIOTARSAL JOINT

INDICATIONS

1. Removal of chip fractures of the medial trochlea of the talus (tibiotarsal bone).[1–3, 5, 6]
2. Surgical curettage and removal of osteochondritic lesions and fragments from the medial trochlea of the talus.[1–3, 5, 6]
3. Surgical removal of chip fractures of medial malleolus of the distal tibia.[1–3, 5, 6]

POSITIONING OF PATIENT

The patient is positioned with the affected limb down.

DESCRIPTION OF PROCEDURE

A. *Topographical View.* A skin incision approximately 8 cm. long is made over the cranial-medial aspect of the tibiotarsal joint, medial to the saphenous vein and fibularis (peroneus) tertius tendon.

B. *Diagrammatic View of Ligaments and Tendons in Relationship to Bones.* The skin incision extends from the level of the medial malleolus of the tibia to the distal border of the medial tendon of the cranial tibial muscle (cunean tendon).

C. *Diagrammatic View of Ligaments, Tendons, and Saphenous Vein in Relationship to Bones.* When the incision is made in the skin and subcutaneous fascia, care should be taken to identify and preserve the saphenous vein, which passes over the cranial aspect of the tibiotarsal joint, medial to the medial border of the fibularis tertius tendon.

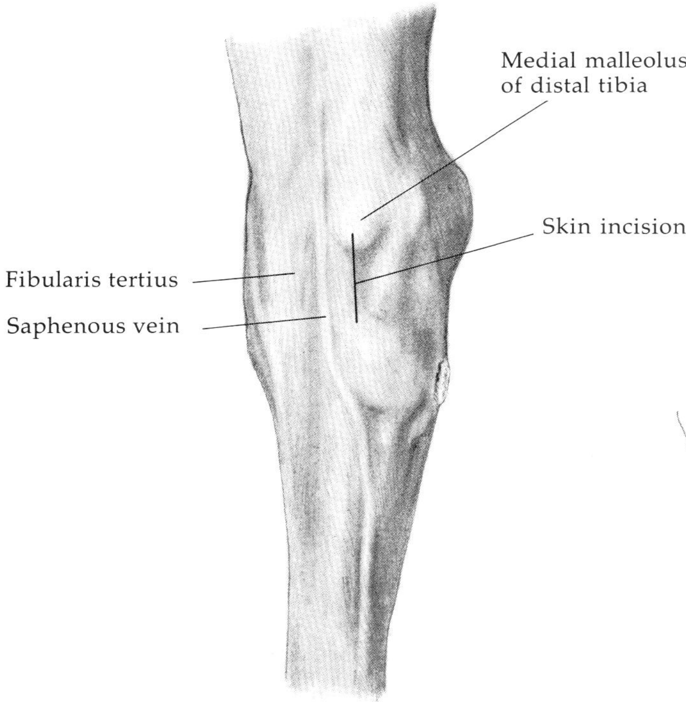
Medial malleolus
of distal tibia
Skin incision
Fibularis tertius
Saphenous vein

A

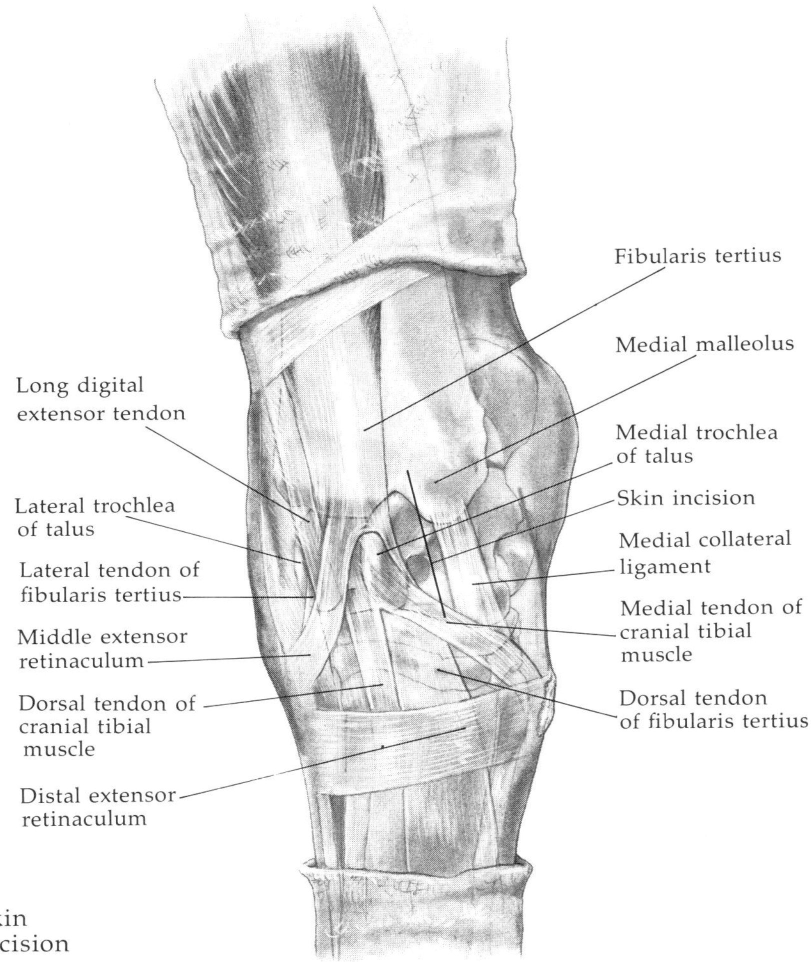
Fibularis tertius
Medial malleolus
Long digital
extensor tendon
Medial trochlea
of talus
Skin incision
Lateral trochlea
of talus
Medial collateral
ligament
Lateral tendon of
fibularis tertius
Medial tendon of
cranial tibial
muscle
Middle extensor
retinaculum
Dorsal tendon of
cranial tibial
muscle
Dorsal tendon
of fibularis tertius
Distal extensor
retinaculum

B

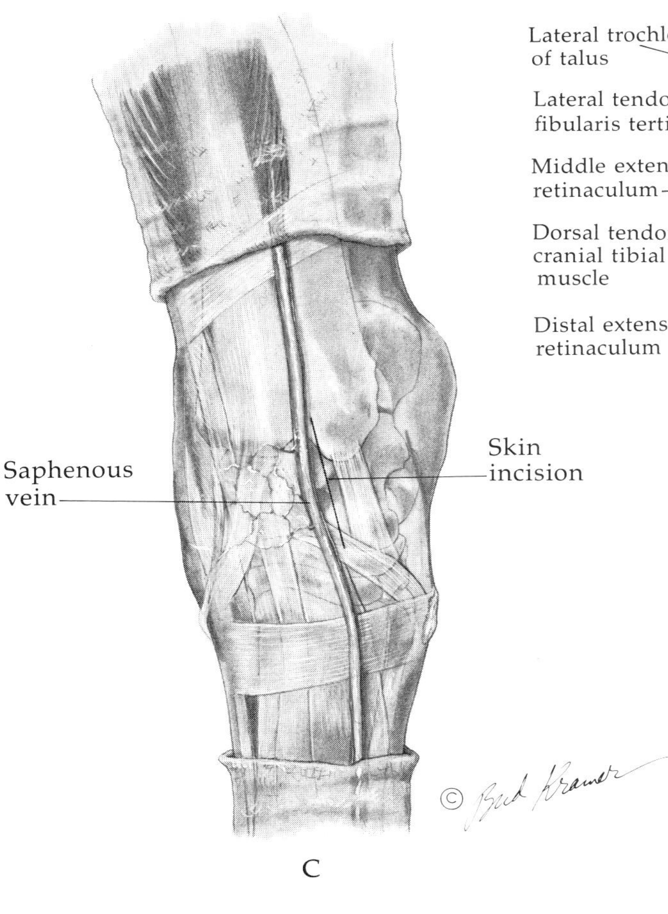
Skin
incision
Saphenous
vein

C

D. *Surgeon's View.* The subcutaneous fascia is incised along the same line as the skin incision. The joint capsule is incised from the distal end of the medial malleoleus of the tibia to the proximal border of the medial tendon of the cranial tibial muscle (cunean tendon).

E. *Surgeon's View.* The medial tendon of the cranial tibial muscle can be retracted to provide greater exposure. The two margins of the joint capsule are retracted laterally and medially as the hock joint is flexed. This exposes the medial aspect of the media trochlea of the talus.

CLOSURE

The joint capsule, subcutaneous tissues, and skin should be closed separately. The sutures in the joint capsule should not penetrate the synovial membrane, nor should the synovial membrane of the joint capsule be allowed to evert between the opposed edges of the joint capsule, as this reduces the rate and strength of healing.[4] Preplacement of the sutures in the joint capsule will allow a more accurate approximation of the cut edges of the joint capsule and achieve a tight seal (each suture is tied after all the sutures have been placed). Interrupted patterns are recommended for closure of the joint capsule. An interrupted or continuous pattern can be used to close the subcutaneous fascia. The skin should be closed with an interrupted suture pattern so that the edges are in firm apposition.

COMMENTS

The cranial-medial approach to the tibiotarsal joint only exposes the articular surface of the medial trochlea of the talus and is not adequate for removal of lesions of the lateral trochlea.

References

1. Birkeland, R., and Haakenstad, L. H.: Intracapsular Bony Fragments of the Distal Tibia of the Horse. J.A.V.M.A. *152*(1968):1526–1529.
2. Carter, E. I., Horney, F. D., and Pennock P. W.: Distal Tibial Fractures in the Horse. Mod. Vet. Pract. (January, 1972):41–42.
3. De Moor, A., Verschooten, F., Desmet, P., and Steenhaut, M.: Osteochondritis Dissecans of the Tibio-Tarsal Joint in the Horse. Equine Vet. J. *4*(1972):139–143.
4. International Symposium of Sutures in Wound Repair. London, England, Ethicon, U.S.A. July, 1972.
5. Schebitz, H., Dammrich, K., Waibl, H.: Intra-articular Fractures of the Hock Joint in Horses. Tierarztl. Wschr. *88*(1975):309–317.
6. Wheat, J. D.: Fractures of the Trochlea of the Tibiotarsal Bone in the Horse. Proc. 100th Ann. Meet. A.V.M.A.:(1963) 86–87.

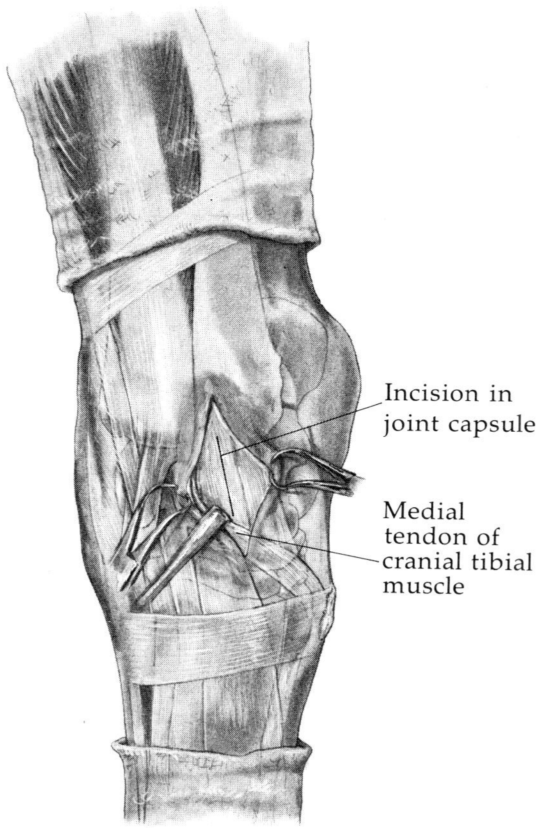
Incision in
joint capsule
Medial
tendon of
cranial tibial
muscle

D

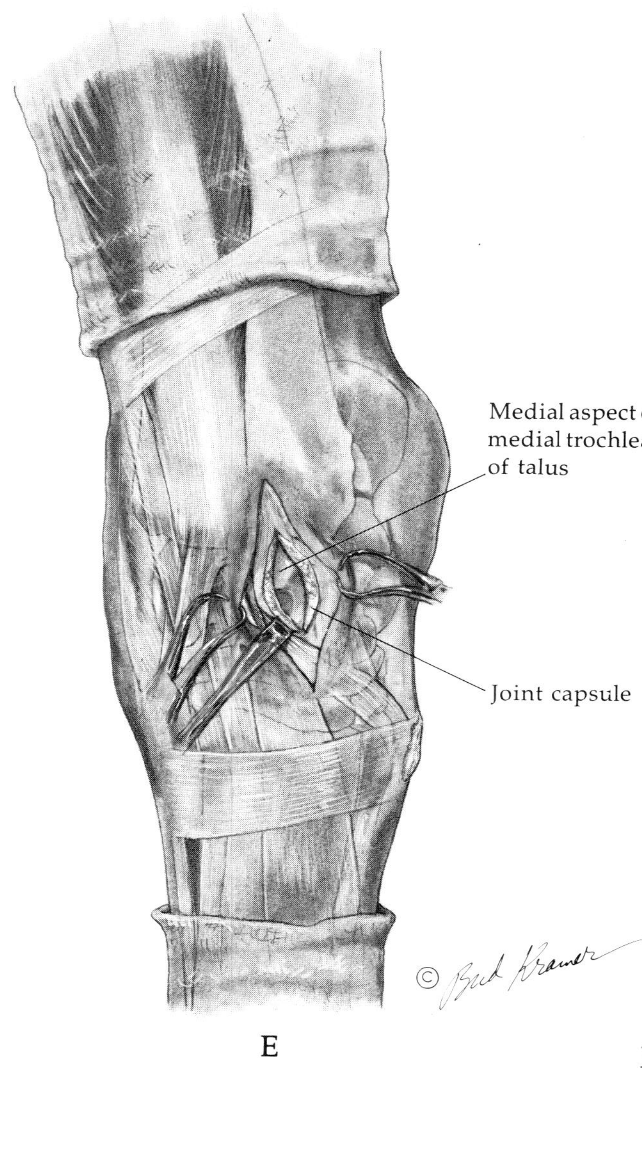
Medial aspect of
medial trochlea
of talus
Joint capsule
© Bud Kramer

E

CAUDOLATERAL APPROACH TO THE CALCANEUS (FIBULAR-TARSAL BONE) AND TUBER CALCIS

INDICATION

1. Open reduction and fixation of fractures of the calcaneus and tuber calcis.

POSITIONING OF PATIENT

The patient is placed with the affected limb uppermost.

DESCRIPTION OF PROCEDURE

A. *Topographical View.* A curvilinear skin incision approximately 20 cm. long is begun from a point approximately 4 cm. proximal to the attachment of the gastrocnemius tendon on the caudal aspect of the calcaneus. The incision arcs over the lateral aspect of the calcaneus with the apex directed laterally, and extends down the caudal-lateral aspect of the bone, in the depression formed by the fascia between the superficial flexor tendon and the plantar ligament. The incision should extend to the level of the head of the fourth metatarsal bone (Mt. IV).

B. *Surgeon's View.* The skin is reflected from the subcutaneous fascia caudally and cranially, exposing the caudal-lateral and lateral aspects of the calcaneus and tuber calcis. The caudal aspect of the calcaneus is covered by the superficial digital flexor tendon and the plantar ligament. The subcutaneous fascia, the capsule of the deep calcaneal bursa, and the tendon sheath of the superficial digital flexor tendon, are incised along the lateral border of the tarsal tendon of the semitendinosus and biceps femoris muscles (accessory tendon), and along the cranial border of the superficial digital flexor tendon, for the length of the skin incision.

CAUDOLATERAL APPROACH TO THE CALCANEUS (FIBULAR-TARSAL BONE) AND TUBER CALCIS

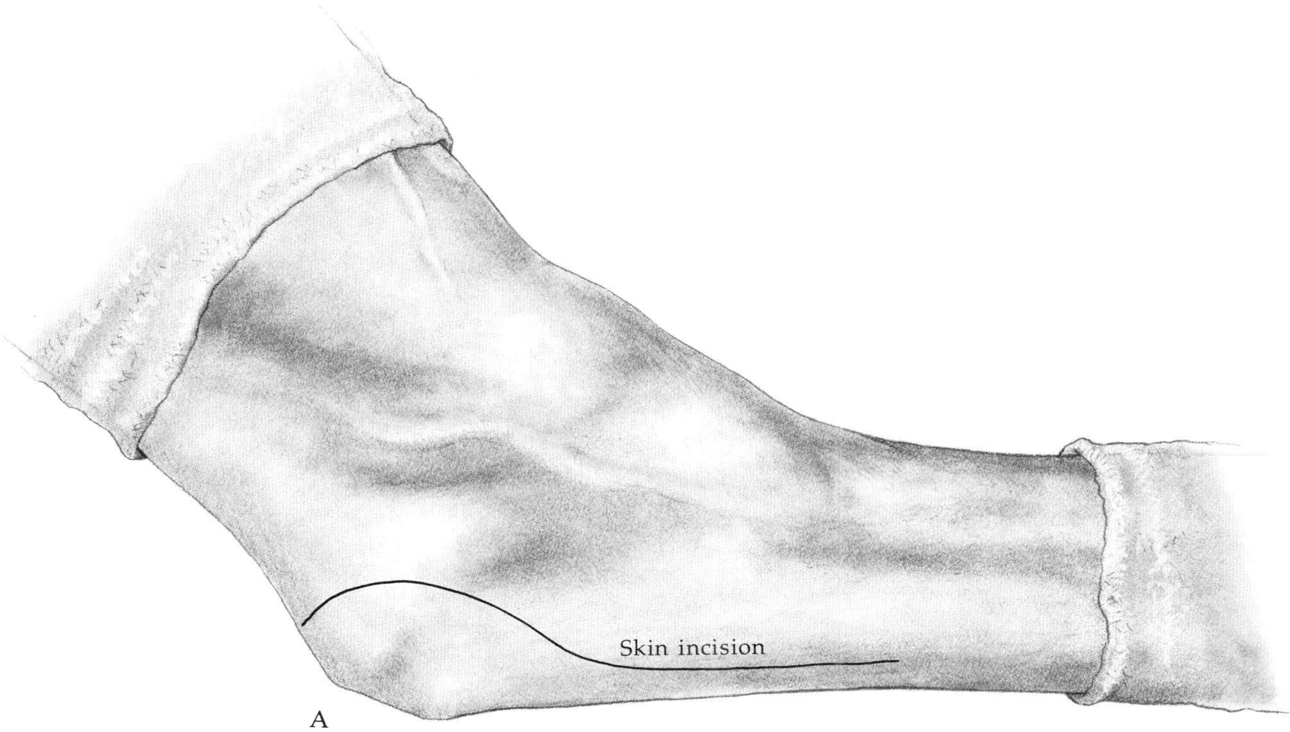

A

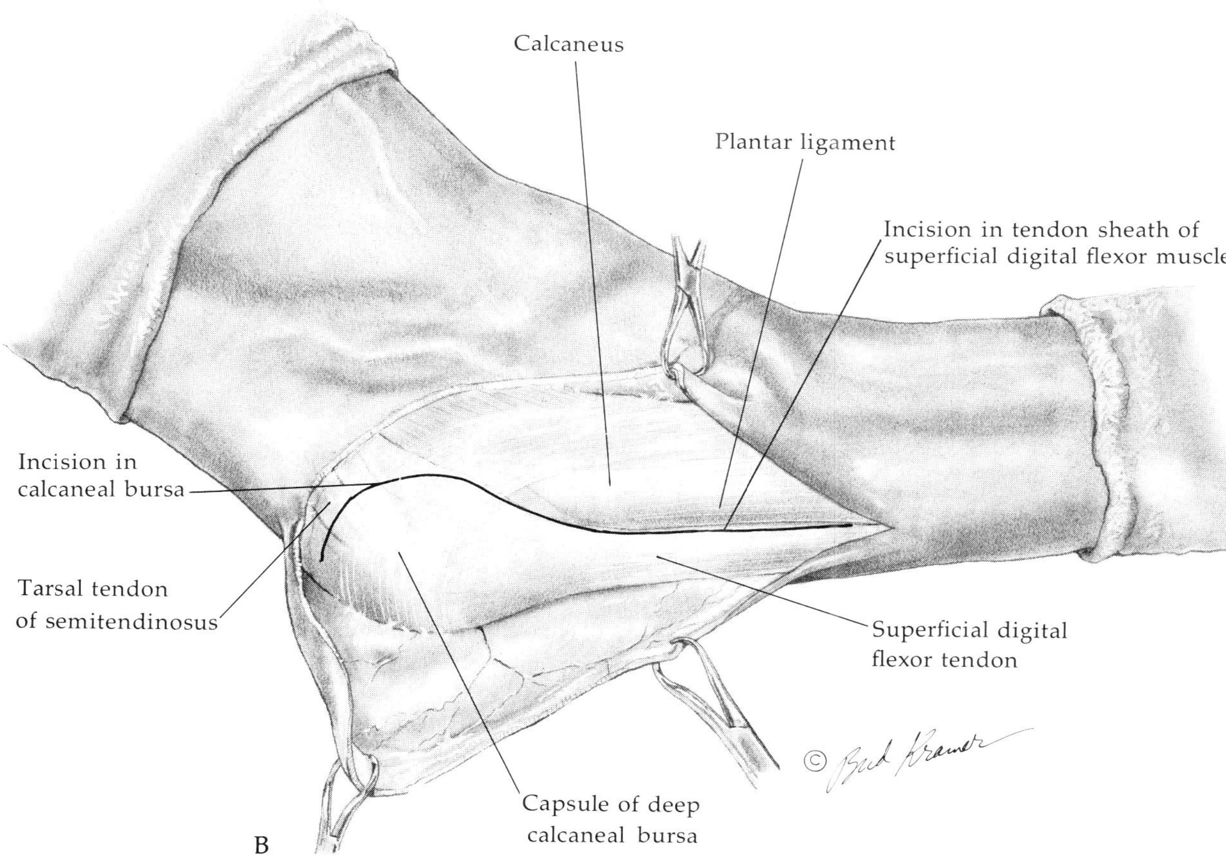

B

C. *Surgeon's View.* This incision will open the deep calcaneal bursa and the tendon sheath of the superficial digital flexor tendon. To expose the caudal aspect of the calcaneus and the tuber calcis, the superficial flexor tendon is luxated medially from its position over the caudal aspect of this bone. Care should be taken to avoid the branches of the caudal-lateral malleolar vein and artery and the lateral plantar cutaneous sural nerve, when reflecting the skin cranially from the subcutaneous fascia (Fig. *D*).

CLOSURE

The fibrous capsule of the deep calcaneal bursa and the sheath of the superficial digital flexor tendon are closed, using an interrupted suture pattern. The subcutaneous fascia is closed using an interrupted or continuous suture pattern. If excessive dead space is present between the bone and the level of the subcutaneous fascia closure, an appropriate drain should be used. This will reduce the accumulation of serum and blood and will help prevent wound dehiscence. The skin should be closed with an interrupted suture pattern so that the edges are in firm apposition.

COMMENTS

Fractures of the tuber calcis are repaired using the tension band principle, with lag screws or bone plates, or both. The tension band side of the calcaneus and tuber calcis is the caudal aspect. This approach allows access to the caudal and lateral aspects of this bone. Placement of the plates on the caudal (tension band side) aspect necessitates placing it under the superficial flexor tendon and over the plantar ligament. This is an advantage from a biomechanical but not from a functional standpoint because of the possible failure of normal function of these structures. Placement of the plate on the lateral aspect is more advantageous from a functional but not from a biomechanical standpoint. The most advantageous placement of the plate at the time of surgery must thus be determined by the configuration of the fracture and the ability to maintain rigid internal fixation.

Reference

1. Ferguson, J. G., and Presnell, K. R.: Tension Band Plating of a Fractured Equine Fibular Tarsal Bone. Can. Vet. J. *17*(12)(1976):314–317.

CAUDOLATERAL APPROACH TO THE CALCANEUS (FIBULAR-TARSAL BONE) AND TUBER CALCIS

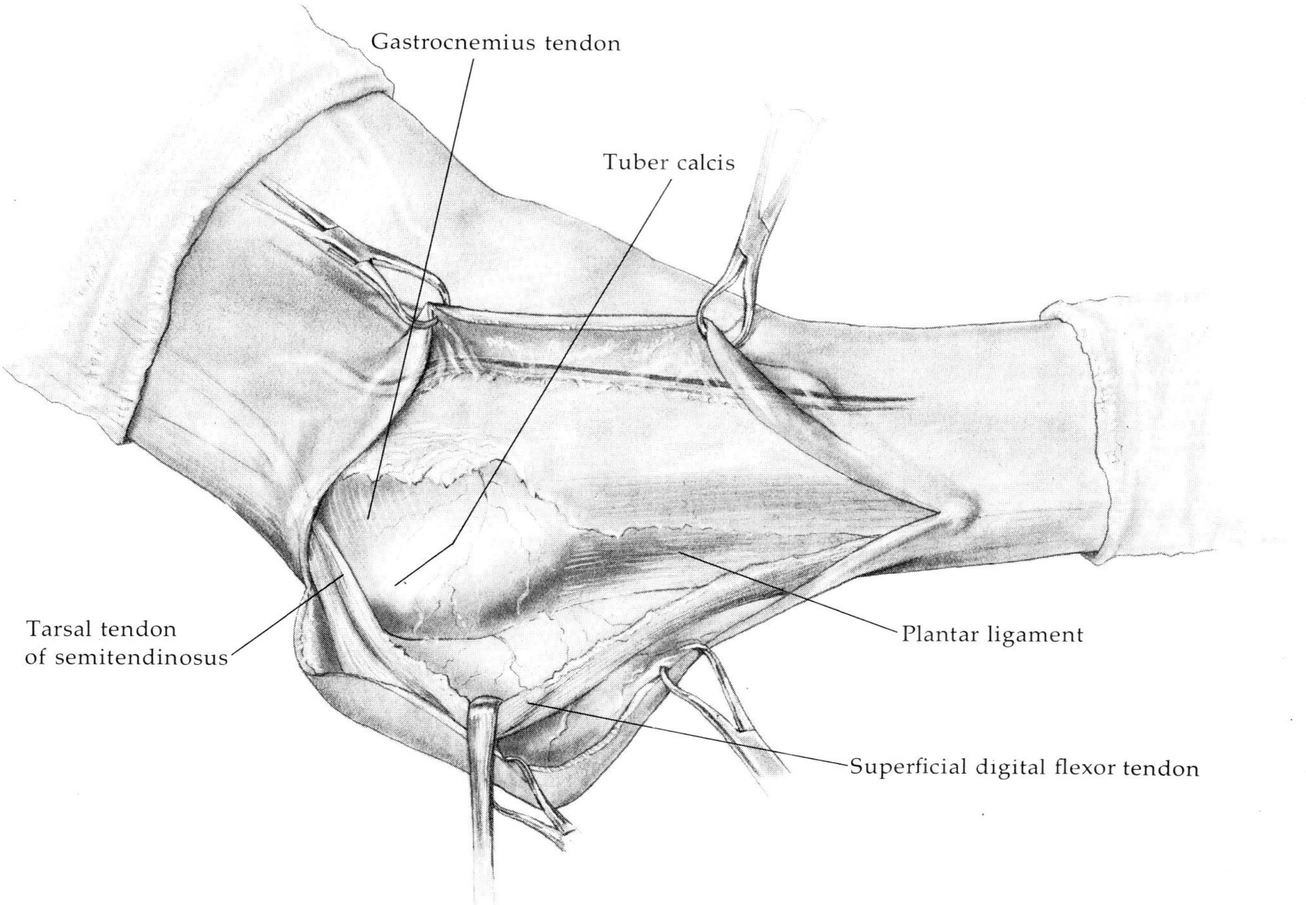

C

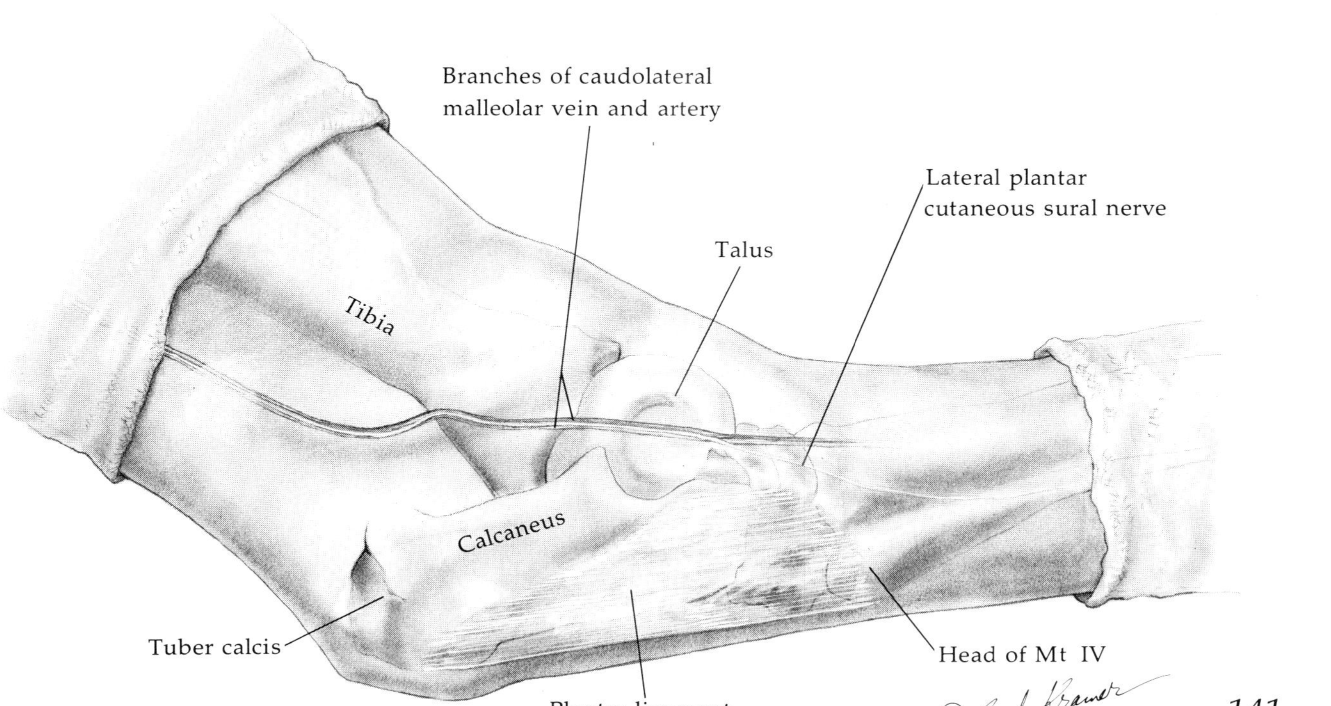

D

part three

Approaches to the Tibia

LATERAL APPROACH TO THE DIAPHYSIS AND METAPHYSES OF THE TIBIA

INDICATION

1. Open reduction and fixation of fractures of the tibia.[1–6]

POSITIONING OF PATIENT

The patient is placed with the affected limb uppermost.

DESCRIPTION OF PROCEDURE

A. Topographical View. A slightly curved skin incision approximately 30 cm. long is made, extending from the lateral condyle of the proximal tibia to the lateral malleolus of the distal tibia. The curve of the skin incision follows the contour of the intermuscular septum between the lateral and long digital extensor muscles.

B and C. Diagrammatic Views. The subcutaneous fascia and intermuscular septum between the lateral and long digital extensor muscles are incised for the length of the skin incision, using sharp dissection. The superficial fibular (peroneal) nerve lies in the intermuscular septum between the long and lateral digital extensor muscles. The deep fibular (peroneal) nerve lies in the intermuscular septum between the long digital extensor muscle and the cranial tibial muscle (Fig. C). These nerves should be identified and preserved.

LATERAL APPROACH TO THE DIAPHYSIS AND METAPHYSES OF THE TIBIA

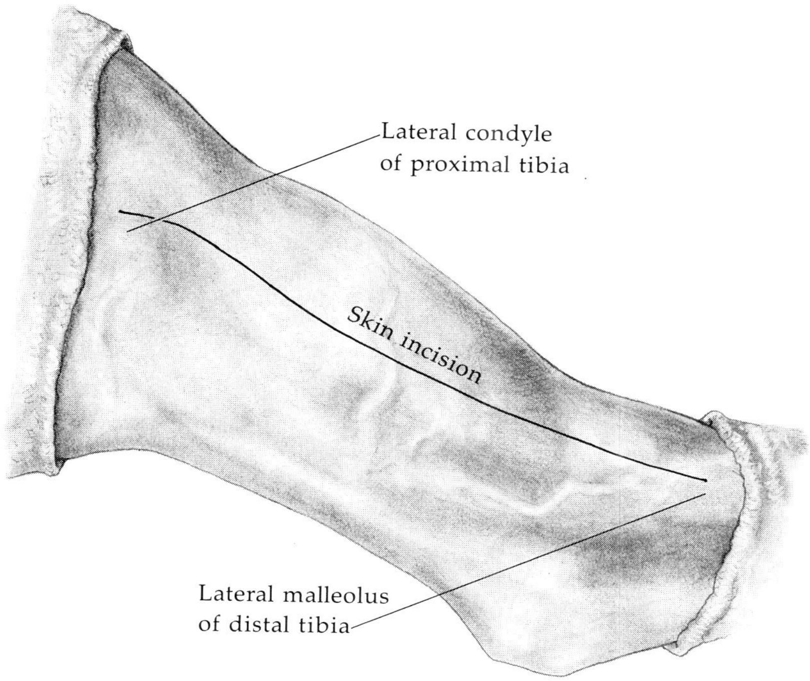

A

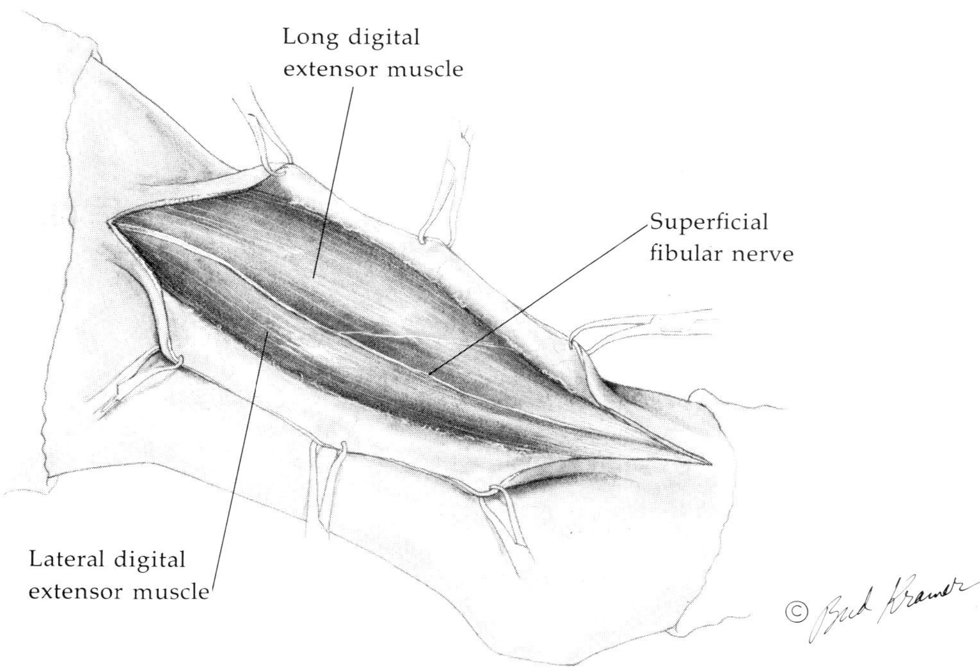

B

D. Surgeon's View. Once the intermuscular septum is incised between the lateral and long digital extensor muscles, blunt finger dissection is used to separate the muscle bellies for the length of the skin incision. To expose the lateral tibia, the long digital extensor muscle and the cranial tibial muscle, which lie deep to it, are retracted cranially. The lateral digital extensor muscle is retracted caudally. The cranial tibial artery and its vein descend on the lateral part of the tibia under cover of the cranial tibial muscle. The artery gives off muscular branches to the cranial group of muscles of the leg. These vessels should be identified and preserved.

CLOSURE

The intermuscular fascial septum and subcutaneous fascia are closed using an interrupted or continuous suture pattern. The skin is closed using a simple interrupted suture pattern with the incised edges in firm apposition.

COMMENTS

This approach is used to place a bone plate on the cranial-lateral aspect (tension band side) of the tibia. It can be used in conjunction with a cranial-medial approach when more than one bone plate is required to establish rigid internal fixation of tibial fractures. Simultaneous medial and lateral incisions will necessitate operating with the horse in dorsal recumbency, with the limb extending upward.

References

1. Alexander, J. T., and Rooney, R. J.: The Biomechanics, Surgery and Prognosis of Equine Fractures. *In* Proceedings, 18th Annual Meeting, American Association of Equine Practitioners, 1972. (1973):219–235.
2. Dingwall, J. S., Duncan, D. B., and Horney, F. D.: Compression Plating in Large Animal Orthopedics. J.A.V.M.A. *158*(1971):1651–1657.
3. Fessler, J. F., and Amstutz, H. E.: *In* Oehme, F. W., and Prier, J. E. (eds.): Large Animal Surgery. Baltimore, The Williams & Wilkins Company, 1974, pp. 309–312.
4. Gertson, K. E., Monfort, J. N., and Tillotson, P. J.: Fracture Repair in Large Animals. Vet. Med. Small Anim. Clin. *68*(1973):782–790.
5. Milne, D. W., Turner, A. S., and Gabel, A. A.: Surgical Approaches to Certain Long Bones of the Horse for Application of Tension Band Plates. J.A.V.M.A. *168* (1976):48–52.
6. Turner, A. S., Milne, D. W., and Gabel, A. A.: The Dynamic Compression Plate in Equine Long Bone Fractures. J.A.V.M.A. *168* (1976):309–315.

LATERAL APPROACH TO THE DIAPHYSIS AND METAPHYSES OF THE TIBIA

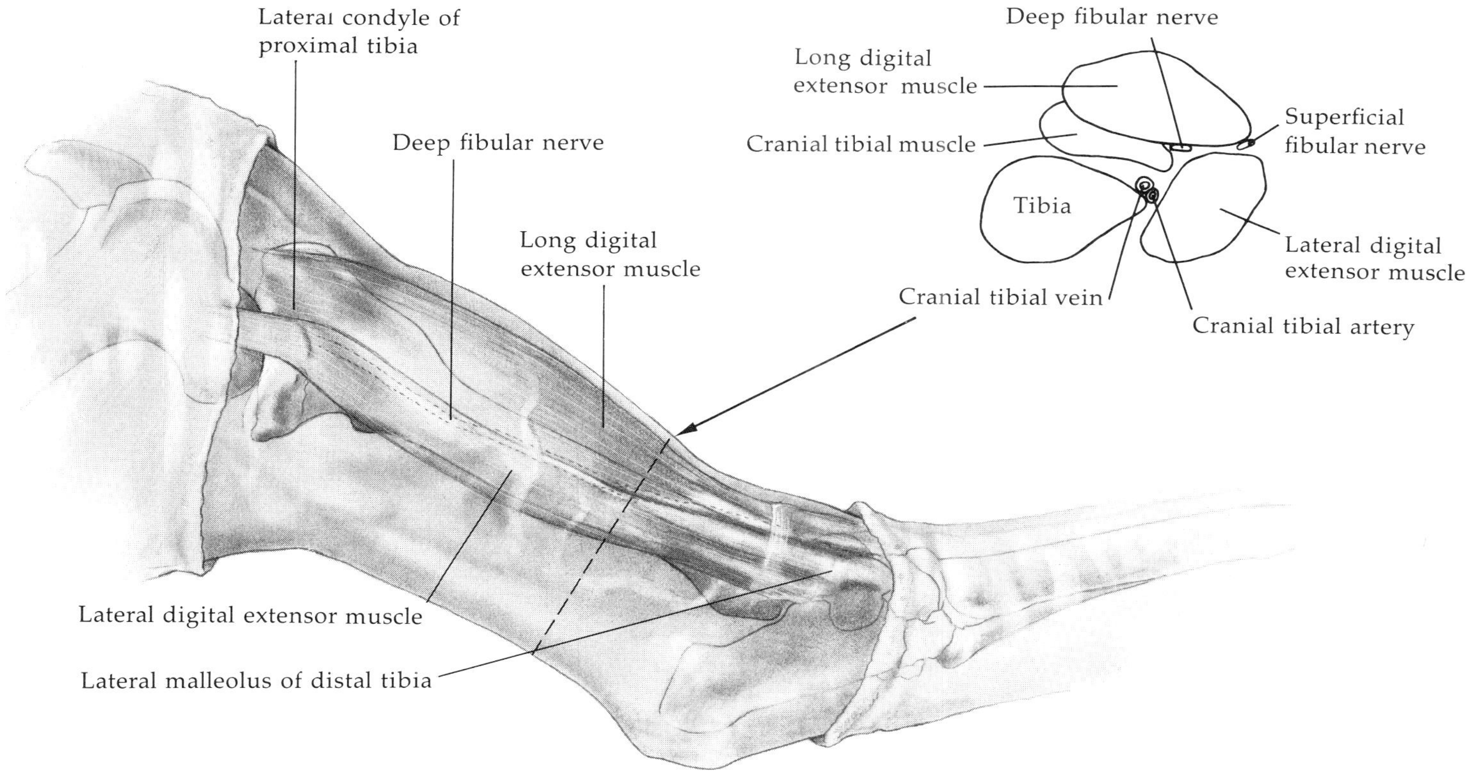

C

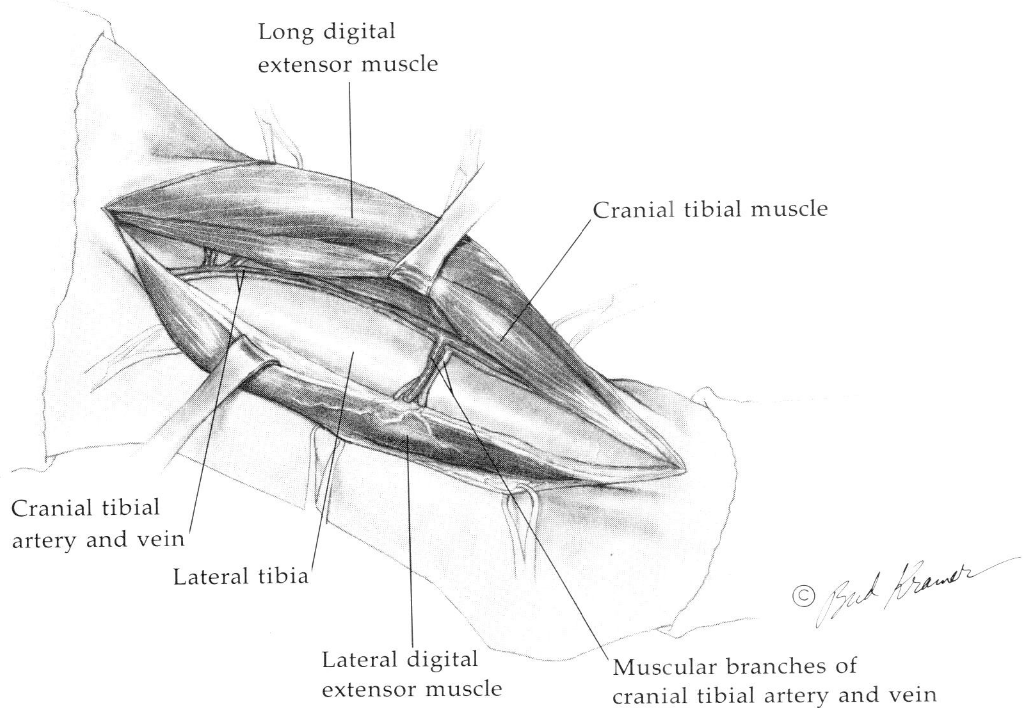

D

MEDIAL APPROACH TO THE DIAPHYSIS AND METAPHYSES OF THE TIBIA

INDICATION

1. Surgical repair of fractures of the radius.[1–6]

POSITIONING OF PATIENT

The horse is positioned in right or left lateral recumbency with the affected limb down.

DESCRIPTION OF PROCEDURE

A. *Topographical View.* A curvilinear skin incision approximately 40 cm. long is made on the medial aspect of the tibia, from the medial malleolus of the tibia to the attachment of the tendon of the sartorius muscle on the medial aspect of the tibial crest. The apex of the skin incision is directed caudally over the medial aspect of the deep digital flexor muscle and the popliteus muscle, and the base of the incison lies cranially over the cranial-medial aspect of the tibia. The skin incision is made carefully, so as not to extend through the medial saphenous vein, artery, and nerve, and the recurrent tibial vein, where they lie between the caudal-medial aspect of the popliteus muscle and deep digital flexor muscle.

B. *Surgeon's View.* The skin is reflected cranially from the apex of the incision toward the cranial-medial aspect of the tibia. The superficial fascia contains the medial saphenous vein, artery, and nerve and the plantar branch of the saphenous vein, which should be left with the superficial fascia when the skin is reflected. A straight incision is made through the superficial fascia over the tibial shaft, extending from the medial malleolus to the border of the tendinous attachment of the gracilis muscle on the tibial crest.

MEDIAL APPROACH TO THE DIAPHYSIS AND METAPHYSES OF THE TIBIA

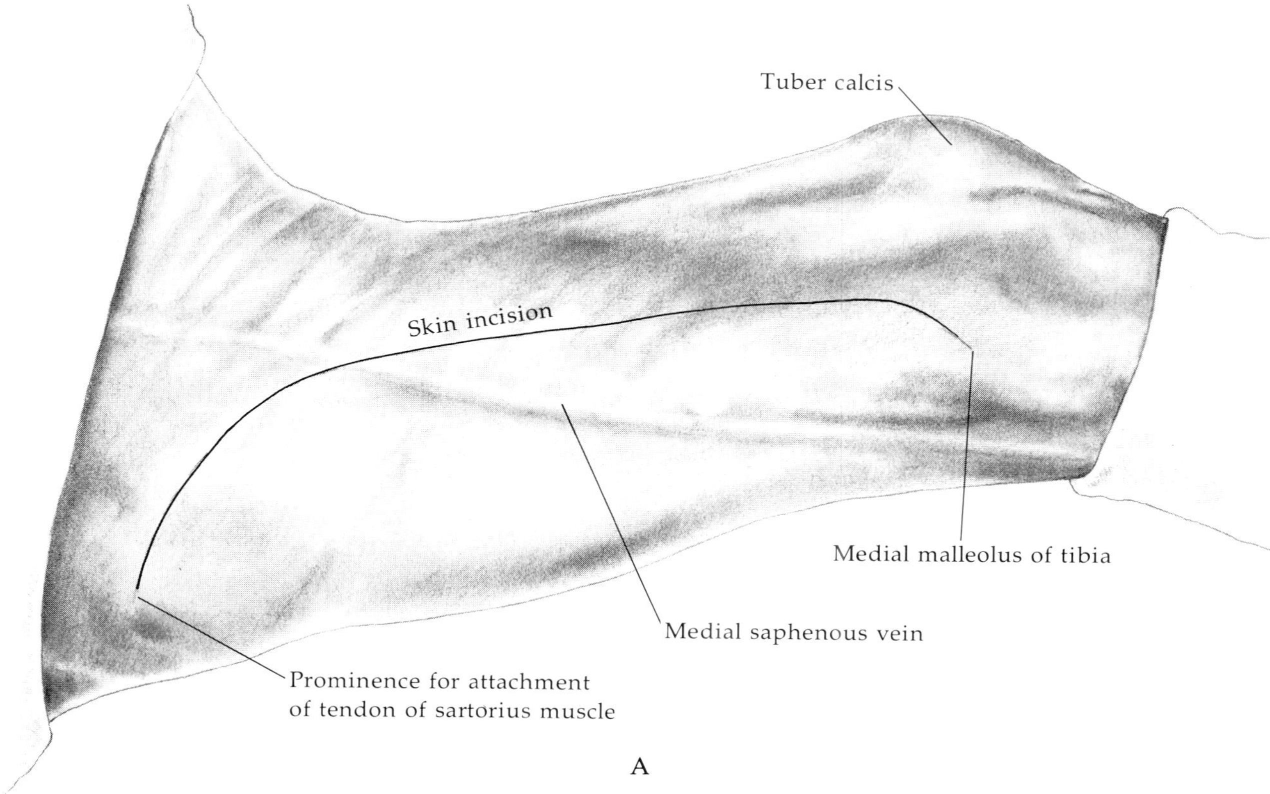

A

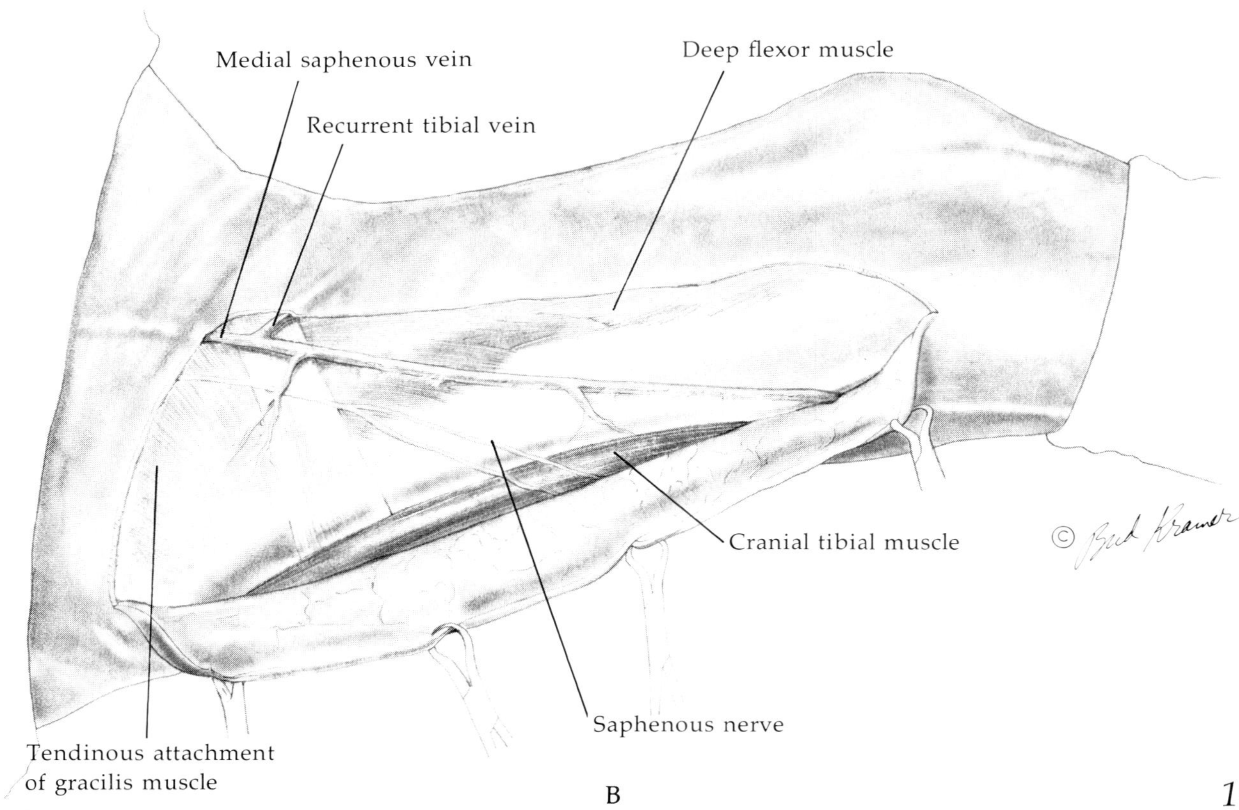

B

C. *Surgeon's View.* The medial saphenous vein and nerve are reflected caudally. An incision is then made through the deep fascial layers of the thigh (fascia cruris), extending from the medial malleolus to the tendinous attachment of the gracilis muscle on the tibial crest. Care must be taken to avoid severing the tibial attachment of the semitendinosus tendon, which lies below the border of the attachment of the tendon of the gracilis muscle. If the more proximal aspect of the tibia needs to be exposed, the fibers of the tendinous attachment of the gracilis muscle are excised to the level of the attachment of the medial collateral ligament of the stifle joint. To apply a plate to the cranial-lateral aspect of the tibia, the cranial tibial muscle is reflected laterally from the tibial shaft. Care is taken to avoid damage to the cranial tibial artery and veins, which lie on the caudal-lateral aspect of the belly of the cranial tibial muscle.

CLOSURE

The subcutaneous fascia is closed using an interrupted or continuous suture pattern. The skin should be closed using an interrupted suture pattern, with the incised edges in firm apposition.

COMMENTS

This approach is used to place a bone plate on the cranial medial aspect of the tibia. It can be used in conjunction with a cranial-lateral approach, when more than one bone plate is required to establish rigid internal fixation of tibial fractures. Simultaneous medial and lateral incisions will necessitate operating with the horse in dorsal recumbency with the limb extended upward.

References

1. Alexander, J. T., and Rooney, R. J.: The Biomechanics, Surgery and Prognosis of Equine Fractures. *In* Proceedings. 18th Annual Meeting. American Association of Equine Practitioners, 1972. (1973):219–235.
2. Dingwall, J. S., Duncan, D. B., and Horney, F. D.: Compression Plating in Large Animal Orthopedics. J.A.V.M.A. *158*(1971):1651–1657.
3. Fessler, J. F., and Amstutz, H. E.: *In* Oehme, F. W., and Prier, J. E. (eds.): Large Animal Surgery. Baltimore, The Williams & Wilkins Company, 1974, pp. 309–312.
4. Gertson, K. E., Monfort, J. N., and Tillotson, P. J.: Fracture Repair in Large Animals. Vet. Med. Small Anim. Clin. *68*(1973):782–790.
5. Milne, D. W., Turner, A. S., and Gabel, A. A.: Surgical Approaches to Certain Long Bones of the Horse for Application of Tension Band Plates. J.A.V.M.A. *168*(1976):48–52.
6. Turner, A. S., Milne, D. W., and Gabel, A. A.: The Dynamic Compression Plate in Equine Long Bone Fractures. J.A.V.M.A. *168*(1976):309–315.

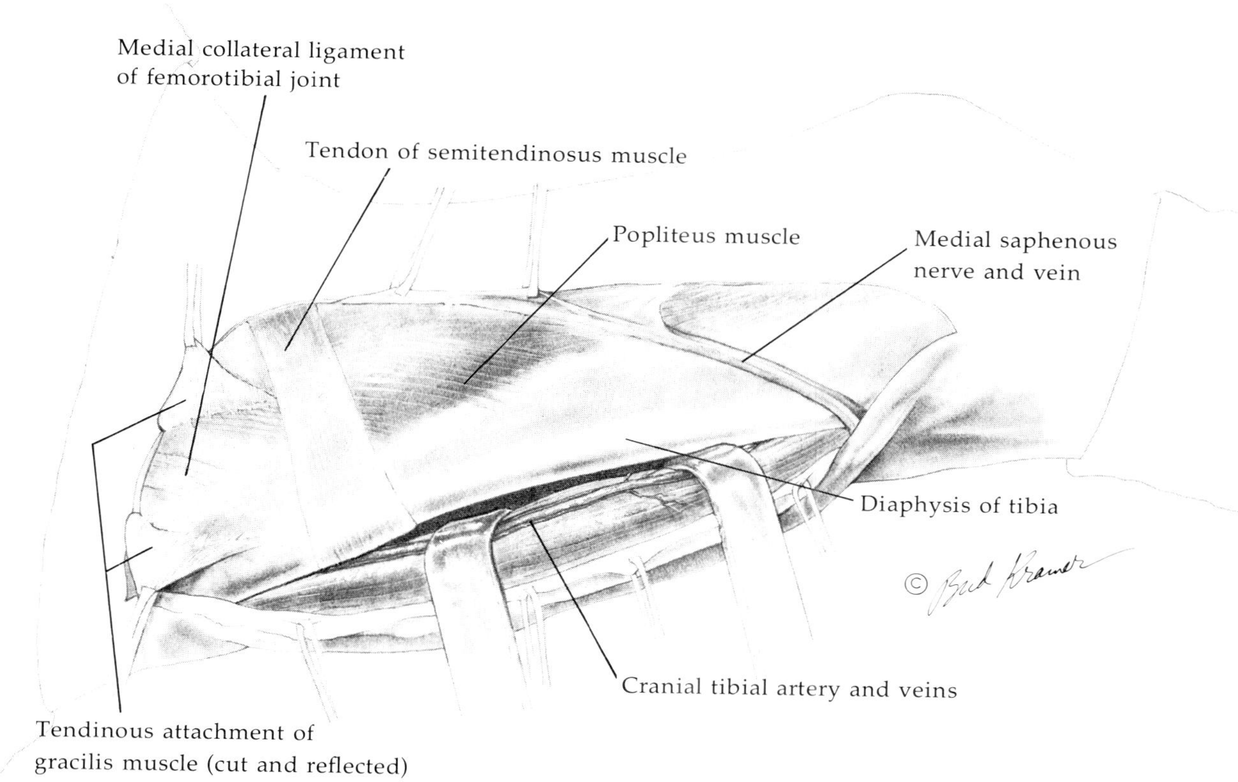
Medial collateral ligament
of femorotibial joint
Tendon of semitendinosus muscle
Popliteus muscle
Medial saphenous
nerve and vein
Diaphysis of tibia
© Bud Kramer
Cranial tibial artery and veins
Tendinous attachment of
gracilis muscle (cut and reflected)

C

part four

Approaches to the Femur

LATERAL APPROACH TO THE DIAPHYSIS AND METAPHYSES OF THE FEMUR

INDICATION

1. Open reduction and fixation of fractures of the femur in the foal.

POSITIONING OF PATIENT

The foal is placed in lateral recumbency with the affected limb uppermost.

DESCRIPTION OF PROCEDURE

A. *Topographical View Showing Underlying Superficial Muscles.* A curvilinear incision approximately 30 cm. long is made, beginning slightly caudal to the greater trochanter and extending to the lateral epicondyle of the femur. The incision lies approximately along the cranial border of the biceps femoris muscle.

LATERAL APPROACH TO THE DIAPHYSIS AND METAPHYSES OF THE FEMUR

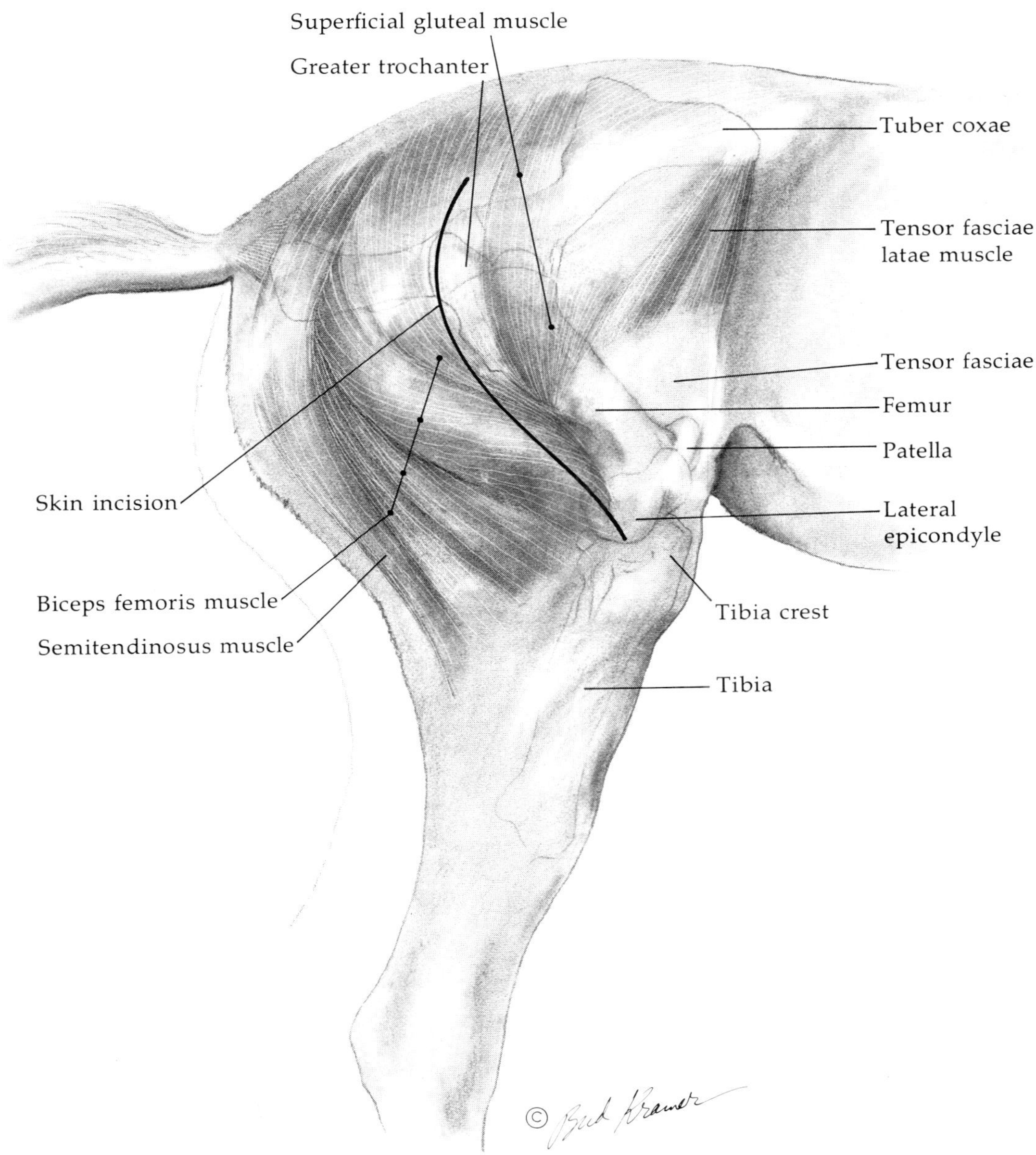

A

LATERAL APPROACH TO THE DIAPHYSIS AND METAPHYSES OF THE FEMUR

B. *Surgeon's View Showing Vastus Lateralis Muscle, Which Lies Deep to the Tensor Fasciae.* The deep fascia is incised in the intermuscular septum between the superficial gluteal muscle and biceps femoris muscle proximally, and the tensor fasciae latae and biceps femoris distally. The attachment of the superficial gluteal muscle to the third trochanter is incised and reflected cranially.

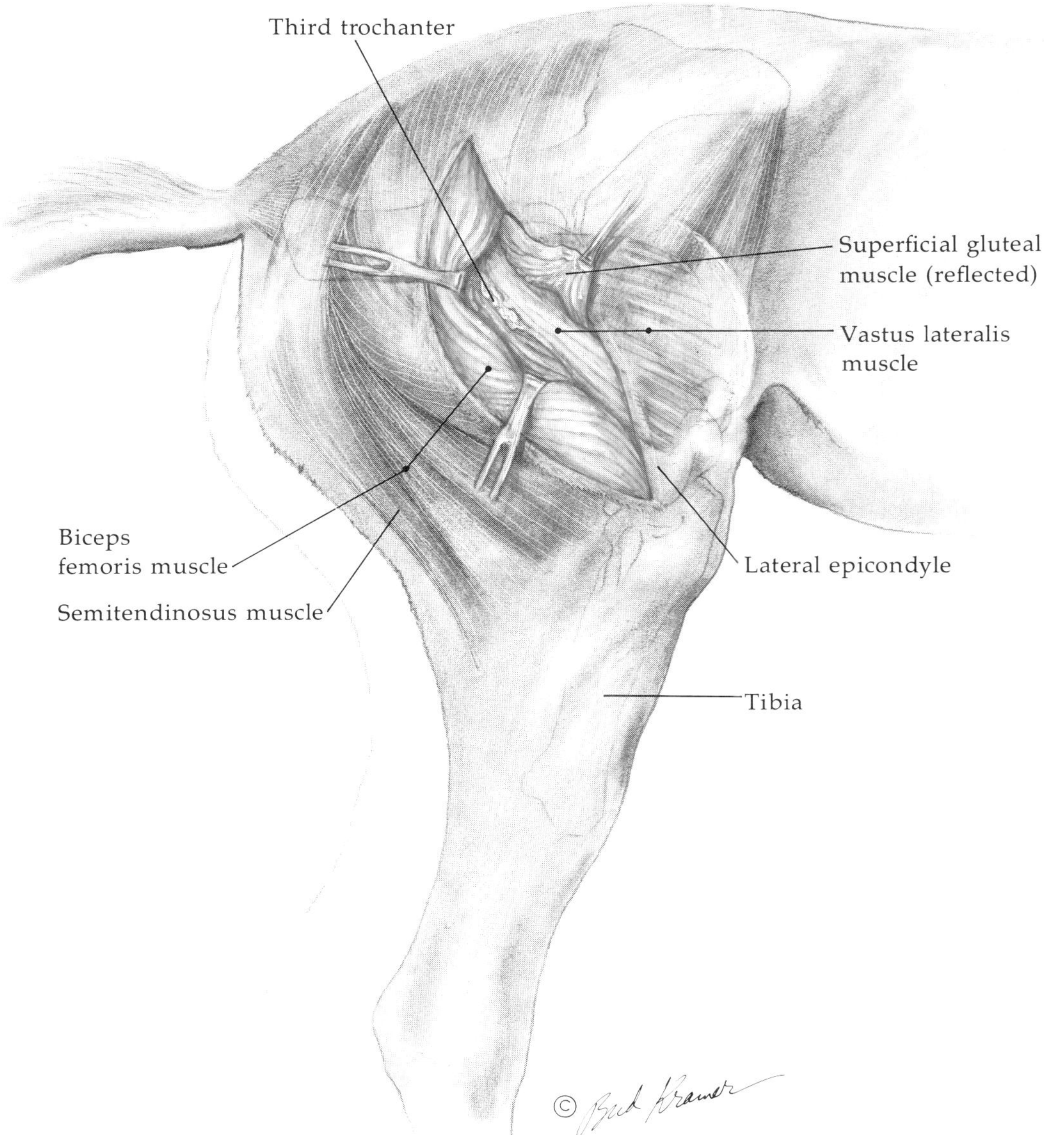
Third trochanter
Superficial gluteal muscle (reflected)
Vastus lateralis muscle
Biceps femoris muscle
Semitendinosus muscle
Lateral epicondyle
Tibia

B

C. Surgeon's View. The shaft of the femur is exposed by retracting the biceps femoris muscle caudally and the vastus lateralis muscle cranially.

CLOSURE

The deep fascia is closed using a simple interrupted or continuous suture pattern. The subcutaneous fascia can be closed using a continuous or interrupted suture pattern. The skin should be closed with an interrupted suture pattern so that the edges are in firm apposition.

Reference

1. Turner, A. S.: Surgical Repair of a Fractured Femur in a Foal: A Case Report. J. Equine Med. Surg. *1*(1977):180–185.

LATERAL APPROACH TO THE DIAPHYSIS AND METAPHYSES OF THE FEMUR

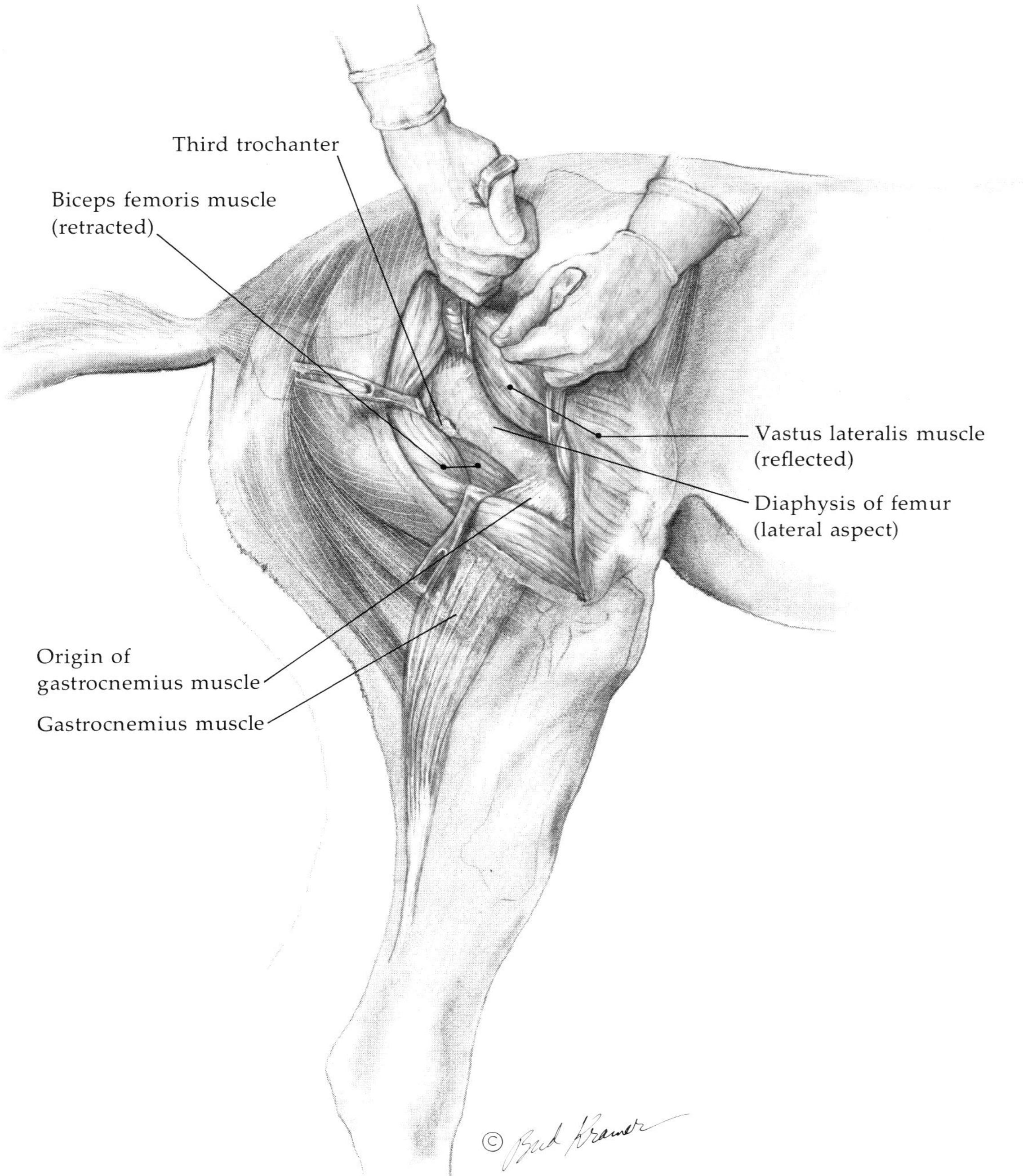

C

DORSAL APPROACH TO COXOFEMORAL JOINT

INDICATIONS

1. Open reduction and fixation of fractures of the head and neck of the femur in the foal.[1]
2. Open reduction of coxofemoral luxations.
3. Femoral head osteotomy and other arthroplastic procedures.

POSITIONING OF PATIENT

The foal is placed with the affected limb uppermost.

DESCRIPTION OF PROCEDURE

A. *Topographical View.* A curvilinear skin incision approximately 26 cm. long is made caudal to the greater trochanter. The incision curves over the biceps femoris muscle and continues distally to the level of the middle of the femur, following approximately the direction of the cranial border of the biceps femoris muscle. The subcutaneous fascia is incised along the same line as the skin incision.

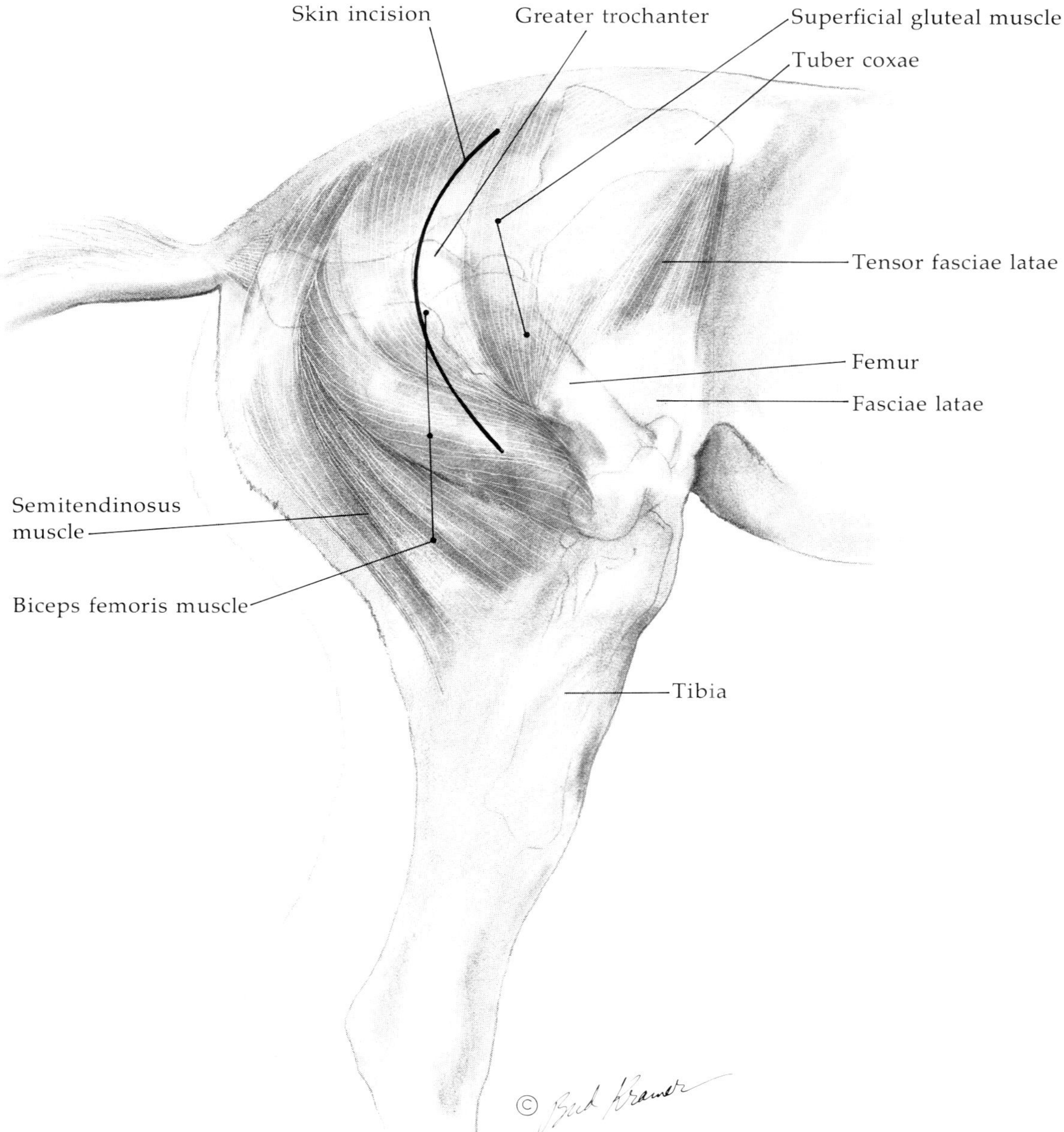
Skin incision
Greater trochanter
Superficial gluteal muscle
Tuber coxae
Tensor fasciae latae
Femur
Fasciae latae
Semitendinosus muscle
Biceps femoris muscle
Tibia

A

B. *Surgeon's View.* The deep fascia is incised along the intermuscular septum between the superficial gluteal and biceps femoris muscles to the middle of the shaft of the femur. This exposes the attachment of the superficial gluteal muscle to the third trochanter. The superficial gluteal muscle is incised from its attachment to the third trochanter and is reflected cranially, exposing the greater trochanter.

The biceps femoris muscle is retracted caudally. When this muscle is retracted, care should be taken to avoid trauma to the sciatic nerve, which lies between the biceps femoris laterally, and the adductor, semimembranosus and semitendinosus muscles medially.

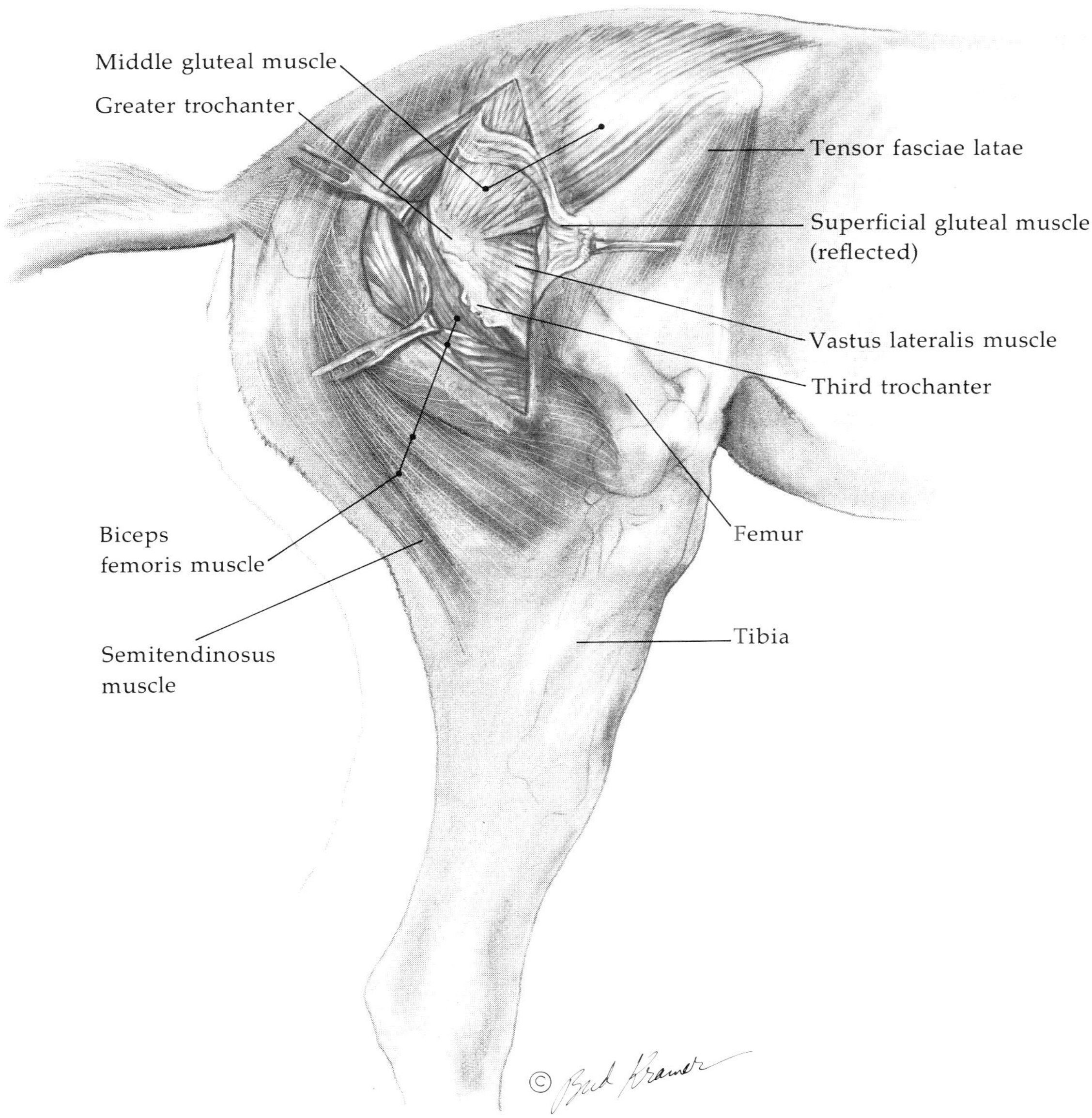
Middle gluteal muscle
Greater trochanter
Tensor fasciae latae
Superficial gluteal muscle (reflected)
Vastus lateralis muscle
Third trochanter
Biceps femoris muscle
Femur
Semitendinosus muscle
Tibia
© Bud Kramer

B

C. Surgeon's View. The deep and middle gluteal muscles are undermined near their attachment to the greater trochanter, and a Gigli wire is passed under their attachments to include as much of the greater trochanter as possible. The greater trochanter is osteotomized and reflected to expose the coxofemoral joint. To visualize the femoral head, the joint capsule is incised.

CLOSURE

The greater trochanter is secured to the shaft of the femur with multiple, partially threaded, cancellous bone screws, with washers. The deep fascia is closed, using a simple interrupted or continuous suture pattern. The subcutaneous fascia is closed, using a continuous or interrupted suture pattern. The skin should be closed with an interrupted suture pattern so that the edges are in firm apposition.

COMMENTS

Prior to osteotomizing the greater trochanter, at least one of the screw holes for reattachment of the greater trochanter should be predrilled. This will allow exact placement of the greater trochanter at closure.

Reference

1. Turner, A. S., Milne, D. W., Hohn, R. B., and Rause, G. P.: Surgical Repair of Slipped Capital Femoral Epiphysis in the Foal. J.A.V.M.A. (submitted for publication).

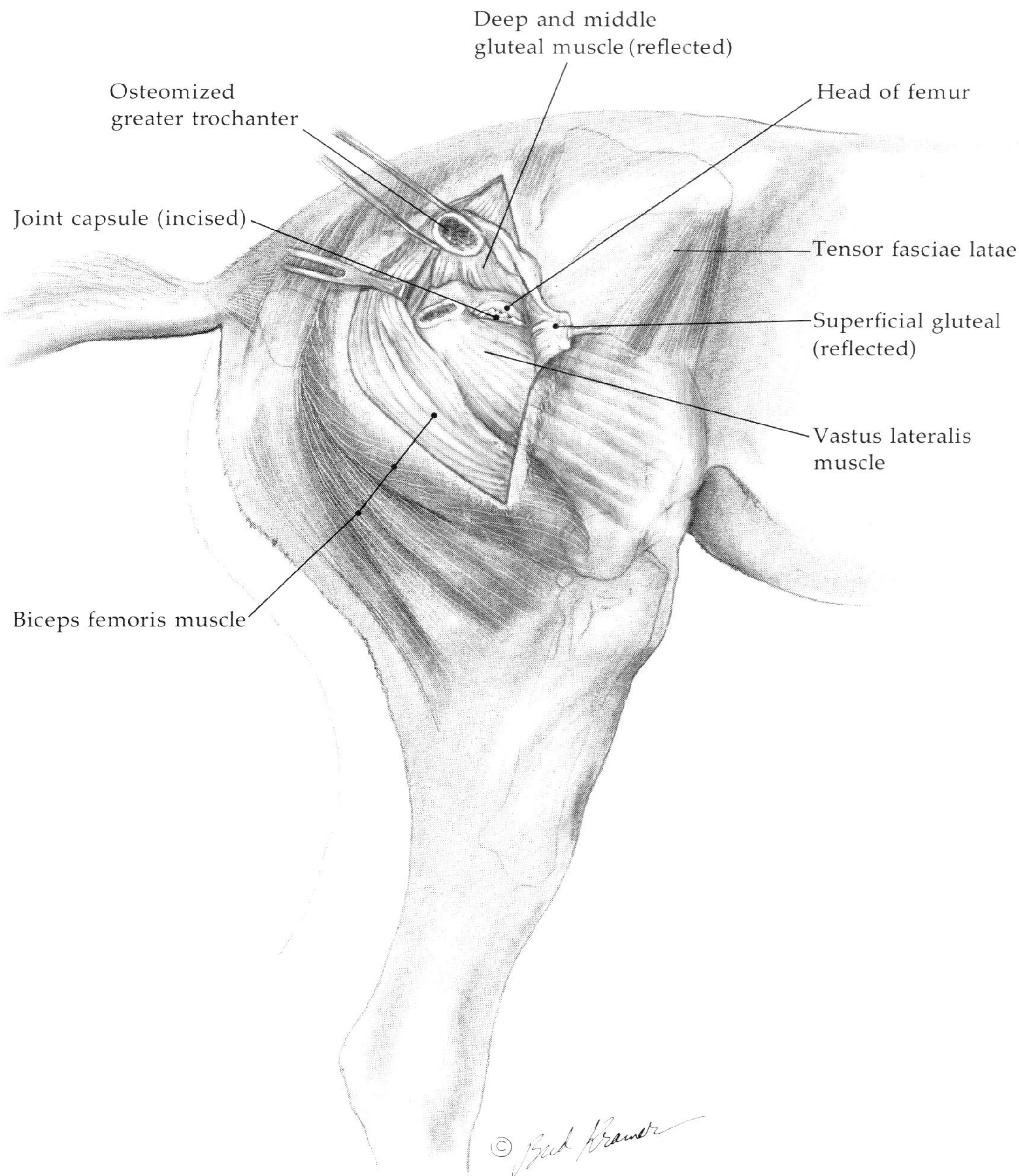
Deep and middle
gluteal muscle (reflected)
Osteomized
greater trochanter
Head of femur
Joint capsule (incised)
Tensor fasciae latae
Superficial gluteal
(reflected)
Vastus lateralis
muscle
Biceps femoris muscle
© Beth Kramer

C

part five

Approach to the Wing of the Ilium

DORSAL APPROACH TO THE TUBER COXAE (GLUTEAL FACE OF ILIUM)

INDICATION

1. Removal of cancellous and corticocancellous bone for autogenous bone grafts.[1, 2]

POSITIONING OF PATIENT

The patient is placed in right or left lateral recumbency.

DESCRIPTION OF PROCEDURE

A. *Topographical View.* A curvilinear skin incision approximately 20 cm. long is made caudal to the tuber coxae with the apex of the incision directed caudally.

B. *Topographical View.* The skin incision is positioned so that it lies over the gluteal face of the ilium. This places the incision so that a rectangular piece of bone can be removed from the gluteal face of the ilium. (Figure supplement)

DORSAL APPROACH TO THE TUBER COXAE (GLUTEAL FACE OF ILIUM)

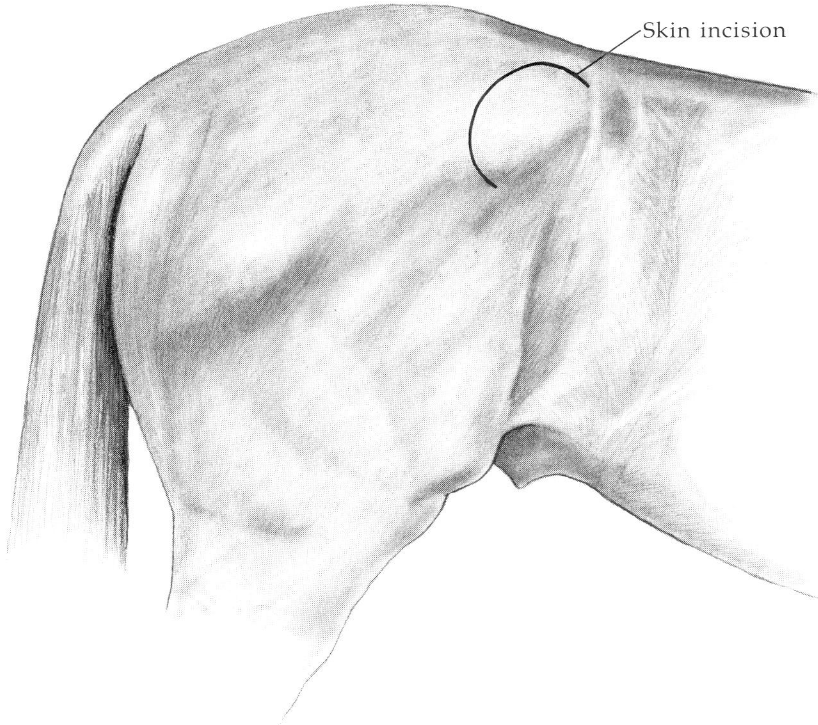

A

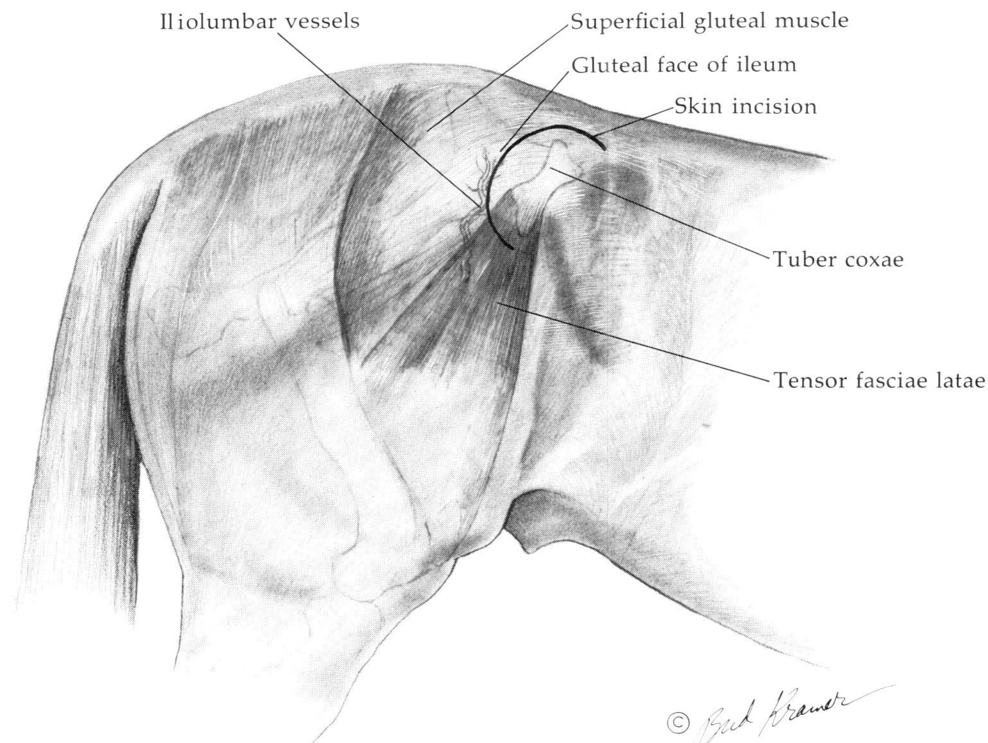

B

DORSAL APPROACH TO THE TUBER COXAE (GLUTEAL FACE OF ILIUM)

C. *Surgeon's View.* The skin incision is reflected from the subcutaneous fascia cranially toward the tuber coxae.

DORSAL APPROACH TO THE TUBER COXAE (GLUTEAL FACE OF ILIUM)

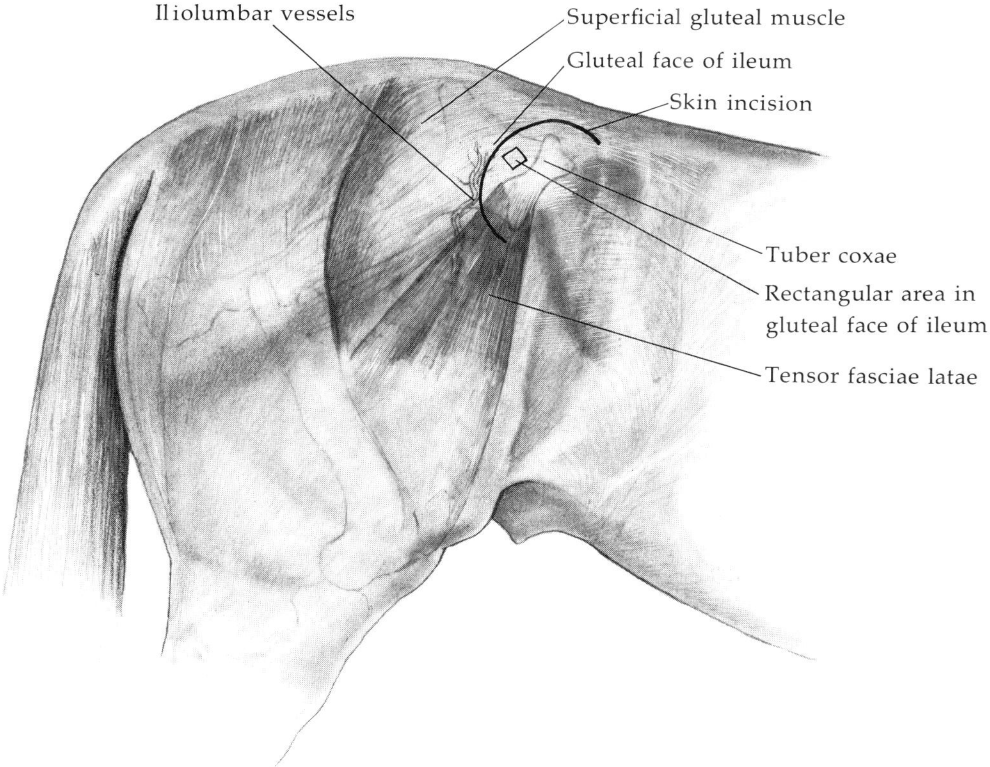

B Cont.

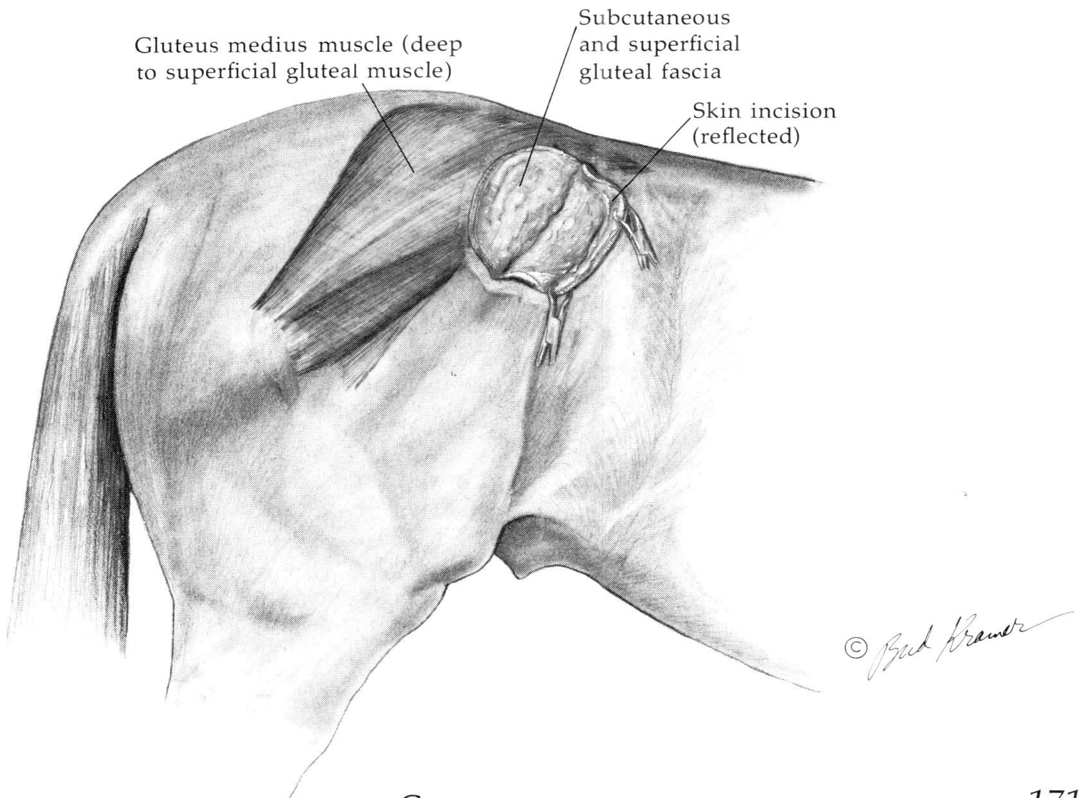

C

D. Surgeon's View. A straight incision is made in the subcutaneous fascia and superficial gluteal fascia.

E. Surgeon's View. The incision is continued deep through the gluteus medius muscle fibers, deep gluteal fascia, and periosteum on the gluteal face of the ilium. The gluteus medius muscle is subperiosteally elevated, revealing the gluteal face of the ilium. Care should be taken not to incise the gluteal muscle too close to the ventral border of the wing of the ilium where the iliolumbar vessels lie (Fig. *B*).

CLOSURE

The superficial gluteal fascia and the subcutaneous fascia are closed together using a simple interrupted suture pattern. The skin is closed with an everting mattress pattern, with the incised edges in firm apposition. A stent suture pattern should also be placed in the skin as tension sutures, to help prevent postoperative wound dehiscence. This is necessary because of excess tension placed on the incision when the horse walks or gets up and down.

COMMENTS

Seroma formation can be a postoperative wound problem if excess dead space is present at closure. A negative pressure or sump drain should be used to prevent serum and blood accumulation to help prevent postoperative wound dehiscence.

References

1. Slocum, B., and Chalman, J. A.: Cancellous Bone Grafts from the Wing of the Equine Ilium: A Surgical Approach. Arch. Am. Coll. Vet. Surg. (Spring 1975):39–45.
2. Stashak, T. S., and Adams, O. R.: Collection of Bone Grafts From the Tuber Coxae of the Horse. J.A.V.M.A. *167,*(1975):397–400.

DORSAL APPROACH TO THE TUBER COXAE (GLUTEAL FACE OF ILIUM)

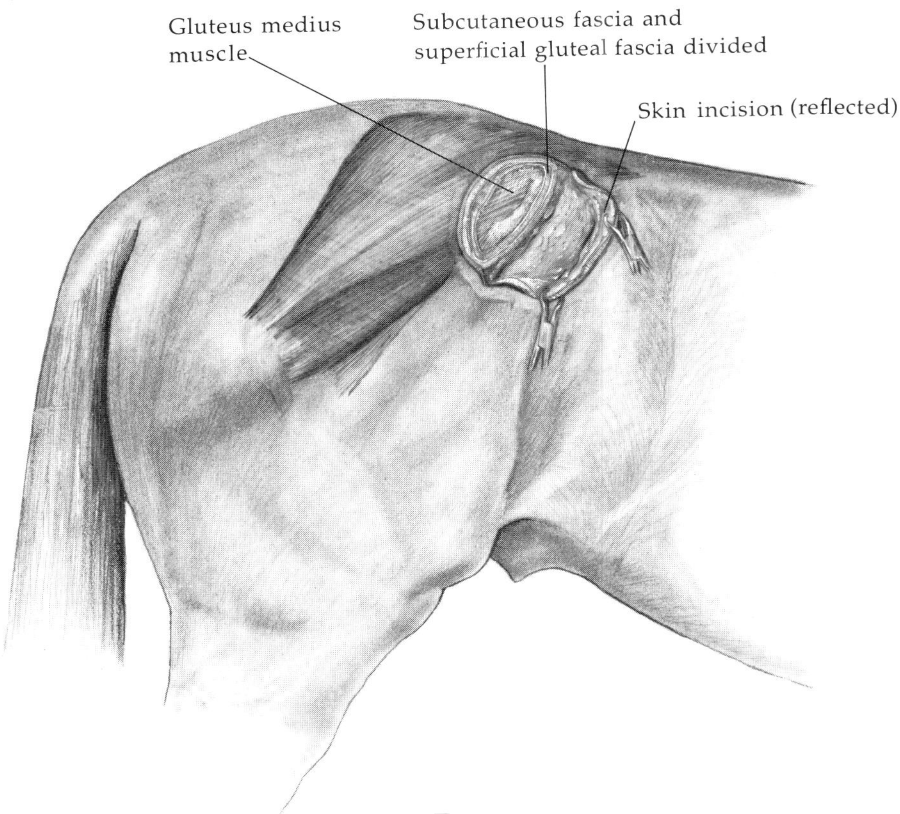

D

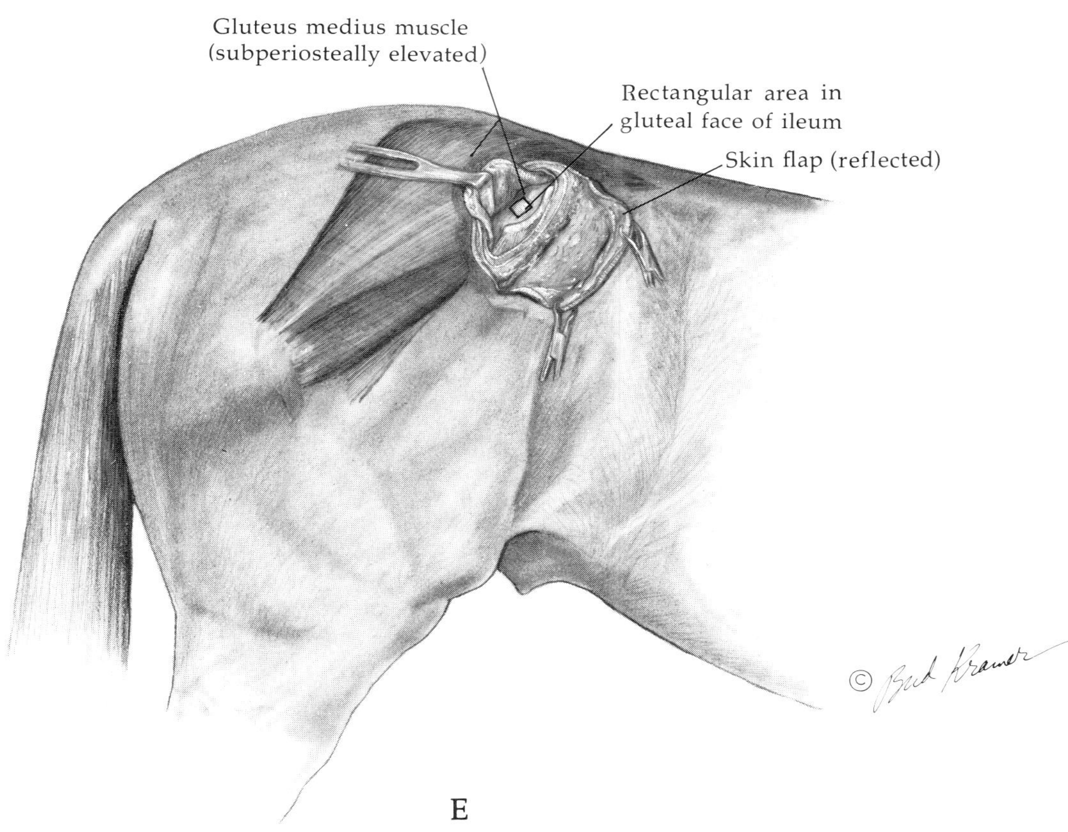

E

section four

HEAD

part one

Approach to the Frontal Sinus

APPROACH TO THE FRONTAL SINUS

INDICATIONS

1. Removal of the upper third molar cheek tooth.[2, 3, 6, 7]
2. Surgical exploration of the frontal sinus for removal of neoplasms, dentigerous and epidermoid cysts, etc.[1]
3. Surgical drainage or curettage of the frontal sinus for frontal sinusitis.[4, 5]

POSITIONING OF PATIENT

The patient is positioned with the affected side uppermost.

DESCRIPTION OF PROCEDURE

A. *Topographical View.* The surgical limits of the frontal sinus are: 1) dorsally, the midline of the forehead; 2) caudally, a line through the supraorbital foramen; and, 3) rostrally, a line perpendicular to the facial crest, halfway between a line through the infraorbital foramen and a line through the medial canthus of the eye. A 7 cm. curvilinear skin incision is made with the apex touching the midline of the forehead (1) and the base parallel to the midline. The incision extends from the caudal (2) to the rostral (3) limits of the frontal sinus.

B. *Surgeon's View.* The apex of the skin incision is reflected from the subcutaneous fascia toward the base. A straight incision is made parallel to the base of the skin incision in the subcutaneous fascia and periosteum, halfway between the apex and the base of the skin incision. The periosteum is reflected with a periosteal elevator, and its two edges are retracted with the subcutaneous fascia, exposing the frontal bone.

CLOSURE

If a large rectangle of bone is removed, it is replaced and stabilized with monofilament stainless steel wire sutures. A trephined hole is usually left to granulate under the soft tissue closure. The subcutaneous fascia is closed using a continuous or interrupted suture pattern. The skin is closed using an interrupted suture pattern with the incised edges in firm apposition.

COMMENTS

To expose the compartments of the frontal sinus and the large nasomaxillary opening, a hole may be trephined through the maxillary bone. To gain greater or wider exposure, the hole can be enlarged by rongeuring around the circumference of the trephined hole. To obtain full exposure of the frontal sinus, a rectangular piece of the frontal bone can be removed by drilling a hole at each edge of the proposed triangle and joining them by cutting with an appropriate cutting instrument. If the surgical procedure is non-aseptic as a result of a procedure requiring entry into the oral cavity (tooth repulsion) or entering an infected sinus, the skin incision may be closed by delayed closure, once infection has subsided or been allowed to granulate in. The authors have found that primary wound healing will be obtained even after non-aseptic conditions have prevailed in most cases. Removal of the sixth tooth is performed by entering the maxillary sinus from the frontal sinus through the nasomaxillary opening.

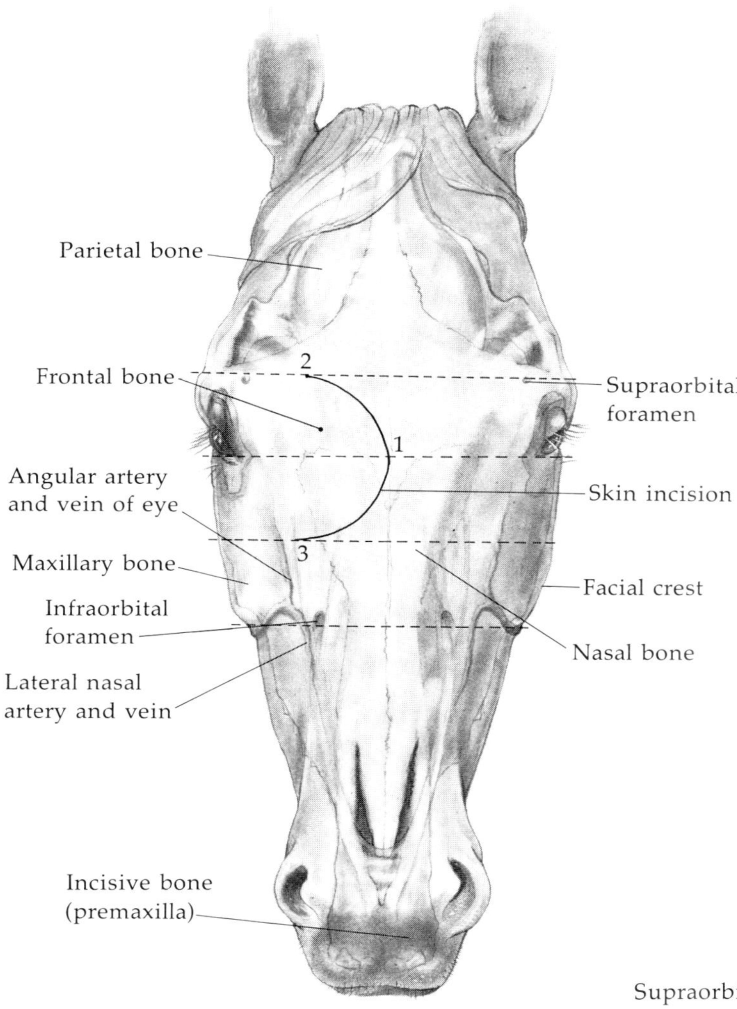
Parietal bone
2
Frontal bone
Supraorbital foramen
1
Angular artery and vein of eye
Skin incision
3
Maxillary bone
Facial crest
Infraorbital foramen
Nasal bone
Lateral nasal artery and vein
Incisive bone (premaxilla)

A

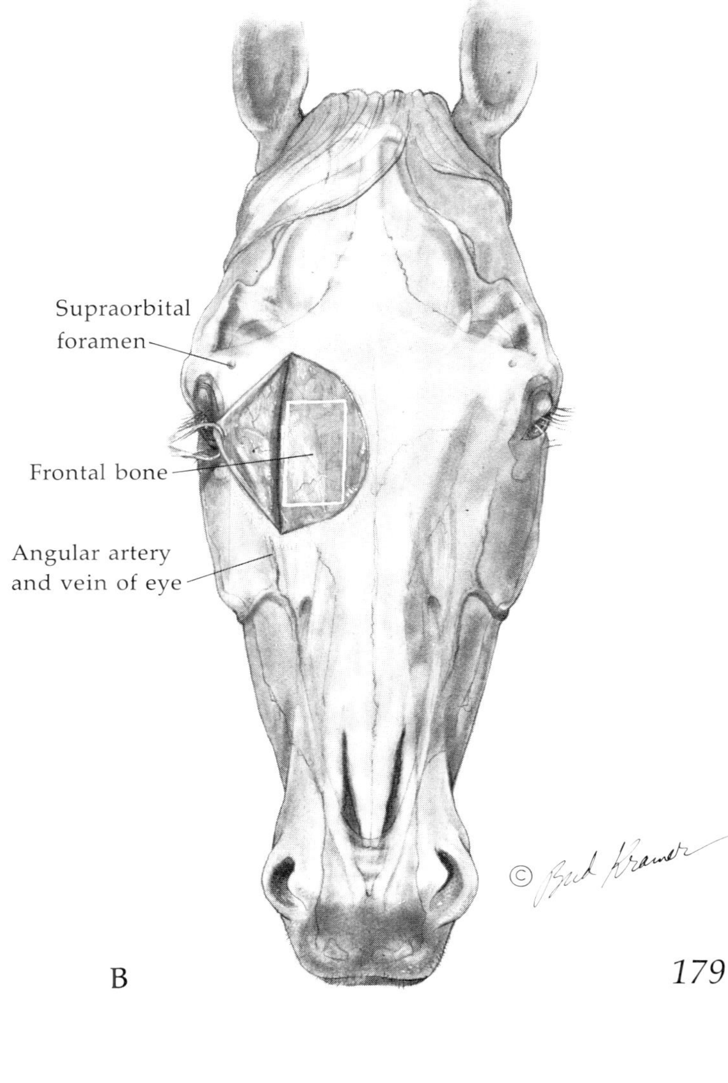
Supraorbital foramen
Frontal bone
Angular artery and vein of eye

B

References

1. Cannon, J. H., Grant, B. D., and Sande, R. D.: Diagnosis and Surgical Treatment of Cystlike Lesions of the Equine Paranasal Sinuses. J.A.V.M.A. *169* (1976):610–613.
2. Cook, W. R.: Dental Surgery in the Horse. Br. Equine Vet. Assn. Bull. (1965/1966).
3. Cook, W. R.: Clinical Observations on the Anatomy and Physiology of the Equine Upper Respiratory System. Vet. Rec. *79* (1966):440–446.
4. Kral, F.: Equine Sinusitis — A New Therapeutic Approach. J.A.V.M.A. *124* (1954):373–376.
5. Mason, B. J. E.: Empyema of the Equine Paranasal Sinuses. J.A.V.M.A. *167* (1975):727–731.
6. Schneider, J. E.: The Respiratory System. *In* Oehme, F. W., and Prier, J. E. (eds.): Large Animal Surgery. Baltimore, The Williams & Wilkins Company, 1974, pp. 348–350.
7. Wheat, J. D.: Sinus Drainage and Tooth Repulsion in the Horse. *In* Proceedings American Association of Equine Practitioners, 1973. (1974):171–176.

part two

Approach to the Maxillary Sinus

APPROACH TO THE MAXILLARY SINUS

INDICATIONS

1. Removal of the third, fourth and fifth upper cheek teeth.[2, 3, 6, 7]
2. Surgical exploration of the maxillary sinus for removal of neoplasms, dentigerous and epidermoid cysts, etc.[1]
3. Surgical drainage and curettage of the maxillary sinus.[4, 5]

POSITIONING OF PATIENT

The patient is positioned in lateral recumbency with the affected side uppermost.

DESCRIPTION OF PROCEDURE

A. *Topographical View.* The surgical limits of the maxillary sinus are: 1) dorsally, a line from the medial canthus of the eye to the infraorbital foramen; 2) ventrally, the facial crest; 3) rostrally, a line from the infraorbital foramen to the rostral edge of the facial crest; 4) caudally, a line from the medial canthus of the eye perpendicular to the facial crest. A 7 cm. curvilinear skin incision is made, with the apex lying just ventral to the angular artery and vein of the eye. The base should extend from the level of the medial canthus of the eye to the rostral limit of the facial crest, parallel and dorsal to it.

B. *Surgeon's View.* The apex of the incision is reflected from the subcutaneous fascia toward the base. Care is taken to avoid the angular artery and vein of the eye, running from the medial canthus of the eye to the anterior edge of the facial crest. A straight incision is made in the subcutaneous fascia and periosteum, lateral and parallel to the levator labii maxillaris muscle.

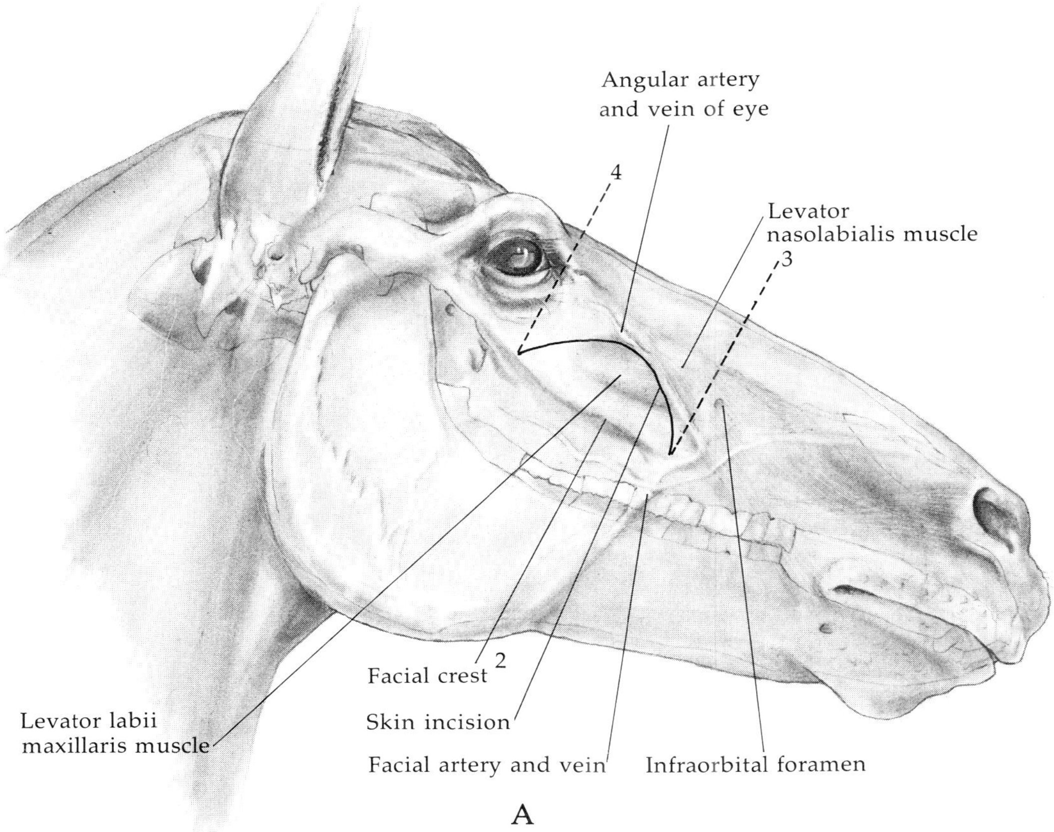
Angular artery
and vein of eye
4
Levator
nasolabialis muscle
3
Facial crest
2
Skin incision
Levator labii
maxillaris muscle
Facial artery and vein
Infraorbital foramen

A

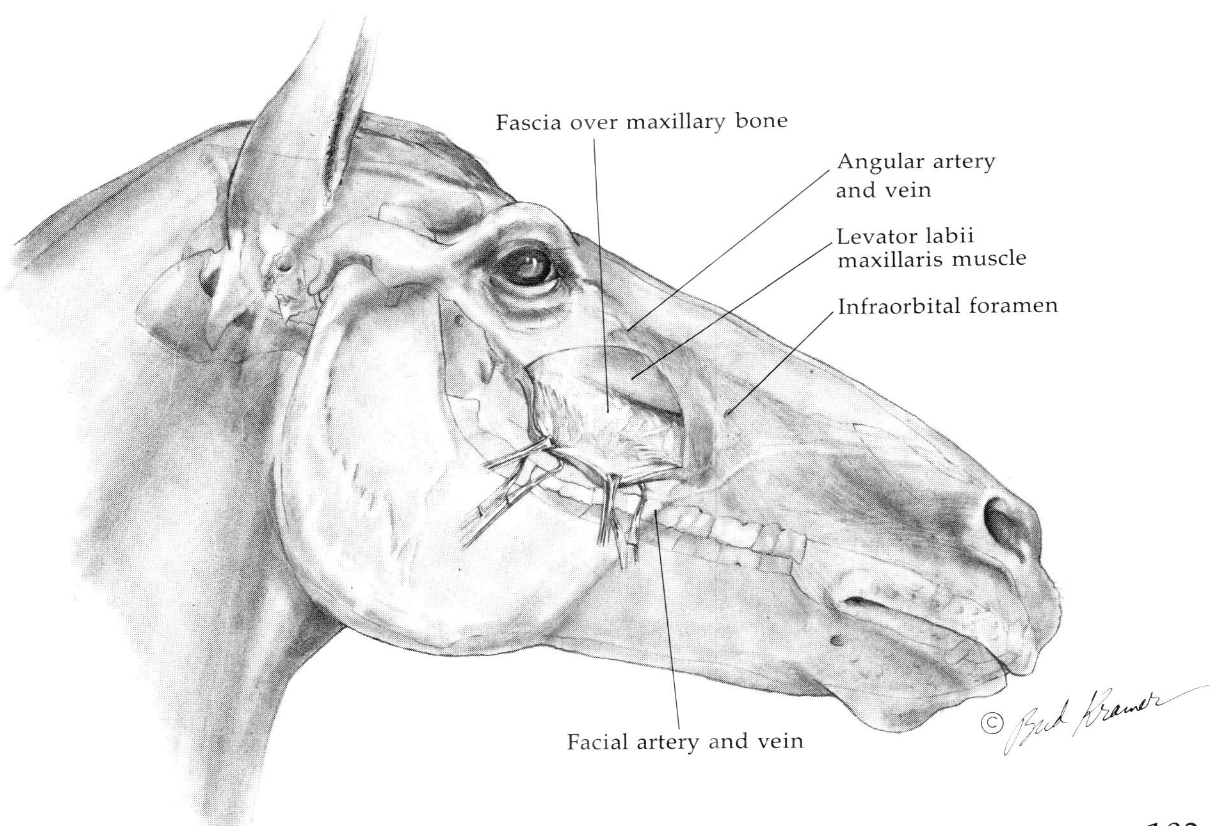
Fascia over maxillary bone
Angular artery
and vein
Levator labii
maxillaris muscle
Infraorbital foramen
Facial artery and vein

B

C. *Surgeon's View.* The levator labii maxillaris is subperiosteally elevated and retracted dorsally, exposing the dorsal portion of the maxillary bone overlying the maxillary sinus. The ventral portion of the maxillary bone overlying the maxillary sinus is exposed by elevating the other incised edge of the periosteum.

CLOSURE

If a large rectangle of bone is removed, it is replaced and stabilized with monofilament stainless steel wire sutures. A trephined hole is usually left to granulate under the soft tissue closure. The subcutaneous fascia is closed using a continuous or interrupted suture pattern; the skin is closed using an interrupted pattern with the incised edges in firm apposition.

COMMENTS

If the surgical procedure is non-aseptic as a result of a procedure requiring the entry to the oral cavity or infected sinus, the skin incision may be closed by delayed closure technique, once the infection has subsided. The authors have found that primary wound healing will be obtained even after infected conditions have prevailed. The maxillary sinus is divided into anterior and posterior parts by an oblique septum. The lateral margin of the septum is commonly about two inches caudal to the cranial end of the fascial crest; from here it is directed inward, backward, and upward. The third, fourth, fifth, and sixth cheek teeth lie in the maxillary sinus. Generally, only the third, fourth, and fifth can be removed from the maxillary sinus. The approach to the frontal sinus must be used to remove the sixth tooth.

To expose the compartments of the maxillary sinus, a hole may be trephined through the maxillary bone. To gain greater exposure, the hole can be enlarged by rongeuring around the circumference of the trephined hole. To obtain full exposure of both compartments of the maxillary sinus, a rectangular piece of the maxillary bone can be removed by drilling a hole at each edge of the proposed triangle, and joining them by cutting with an appropriate cutting instrument.

References

1. Cannon, J. H., Grant, B. D., and Sande, R. D.: Diagnosis and Surgical Treatment of Cystlike Lesions of the Equine Paranasal Sinuses. J.A.V.M.A. *169* (1976):610–613.
2. Cook, W. R.: Dental Surgery in the Horse. Br. Equine Vet. Assn. Bull. (1965/1966).
3. Cook, W. R.: Clinical Observations on the Anatomy and Physiology of the Equine Upper Respiratory System. Vet. Rec. *79* (1966):440–446.
4. Kral, F.: Equine Sinusitis — A New Therapeutic Approach. J.A.V.M.A. *124* (1954):373–376.
5. Mason, B. J. E.: Empyema of the Equine Paranasal Sinuses. J.A.V.M.A. *167* (1975):727–731.
6. Schneider, J. E.: The Respiratory System. *In* Oehme, F. W., and Prier, J. E. (eds.): Large Animal Surery. Baltimore, The Williams & Wilkins Company, 1974, pp. 348–350.
7. Wheat, J. D.: Sinus Drainage and Tooth Repulsion in the Horse. *In* Proceedings American Association of Equine Practitioners, 1973. (1974):171–176.

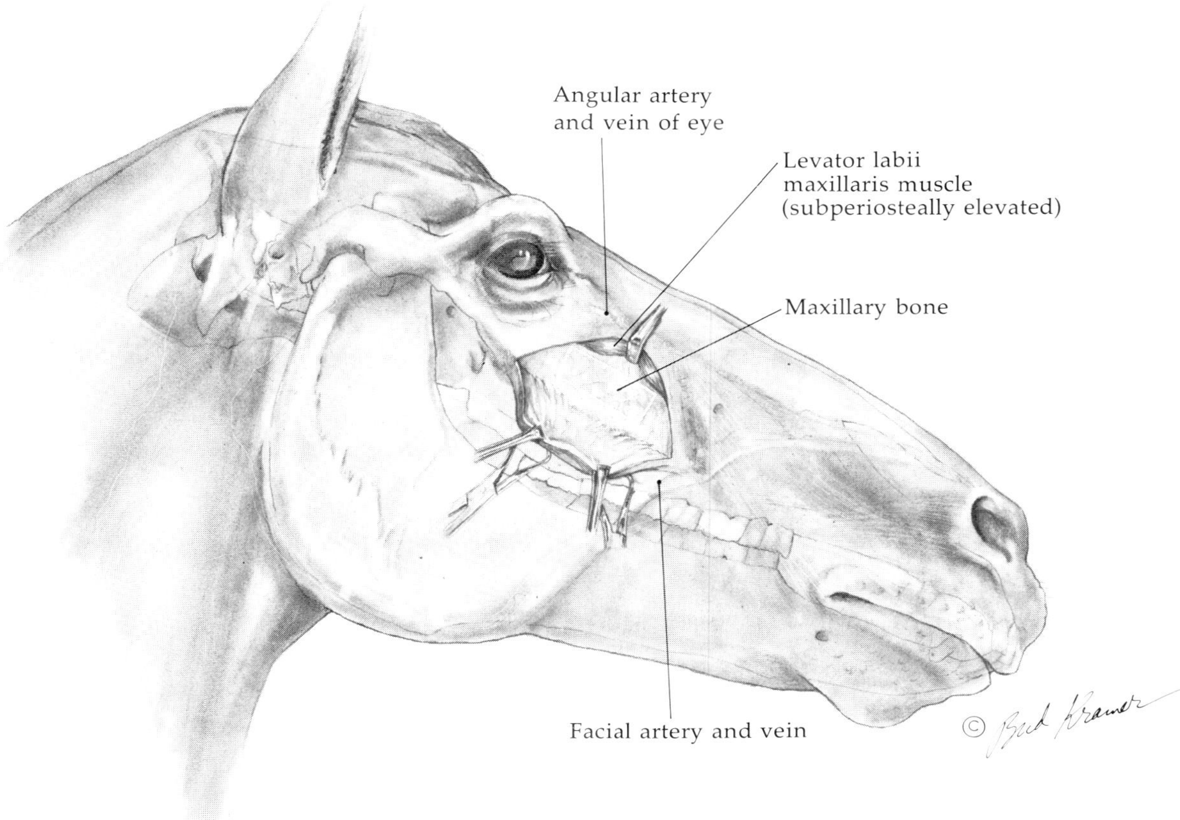
Angular artery
and vein of eye
Levator labii
maxillaris muscle
(subperiosteally elevated)
Maxillary bone
Facial artery and vein
© Bud Kramer

C

part three

Approach to the Horizontal Ramus of the Mandible

LATERAL APPROACH TO THE HORIZONTAL RAMUS OF THE MANDIBLE

INDICATION

1. Open reduction and fixation of fractures of the mandible.

POSITIONING OF PATIENT

The patient is positioned with the affected side uppermost.

DESCRIPTION OF PROCEDURE

A. Topographical View. A skin incision approximately 14 cm. long is made along the ventral-lateral aspect of the horizontal ramus of the mandible, extending from the level of the commissure of the lips to the cranial edge of the masseter muscle.

B. Surgeon's View. The subcutaneous fascia is incised along the same line as the skin incision. Care should be taken to identify and preserve the parotid duct and the facial artery and vein, which pass along the cranial edge of the masseter muscle. The mental nerve should also be preserved as it emerges from the mental foramen.

LATERAL APPROACH TO THE HORIZONTAL RAMUS OF THE MANDIBLE

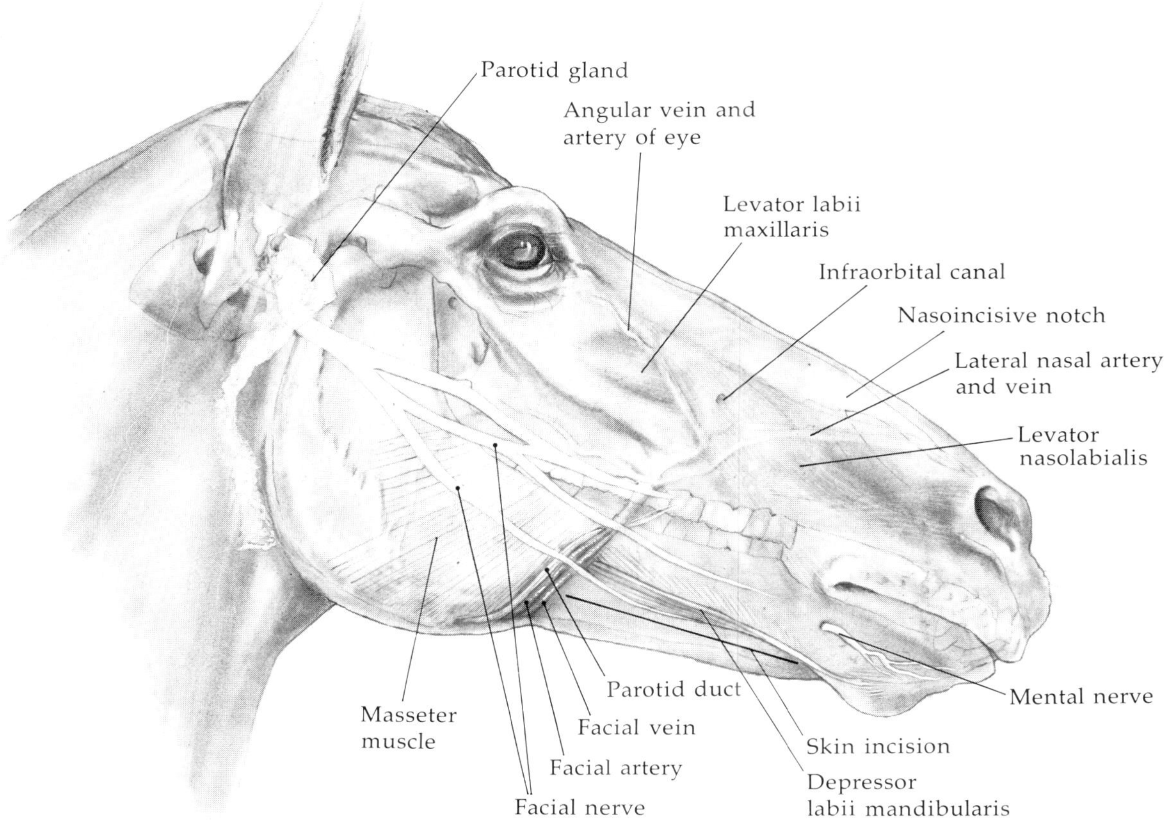

A

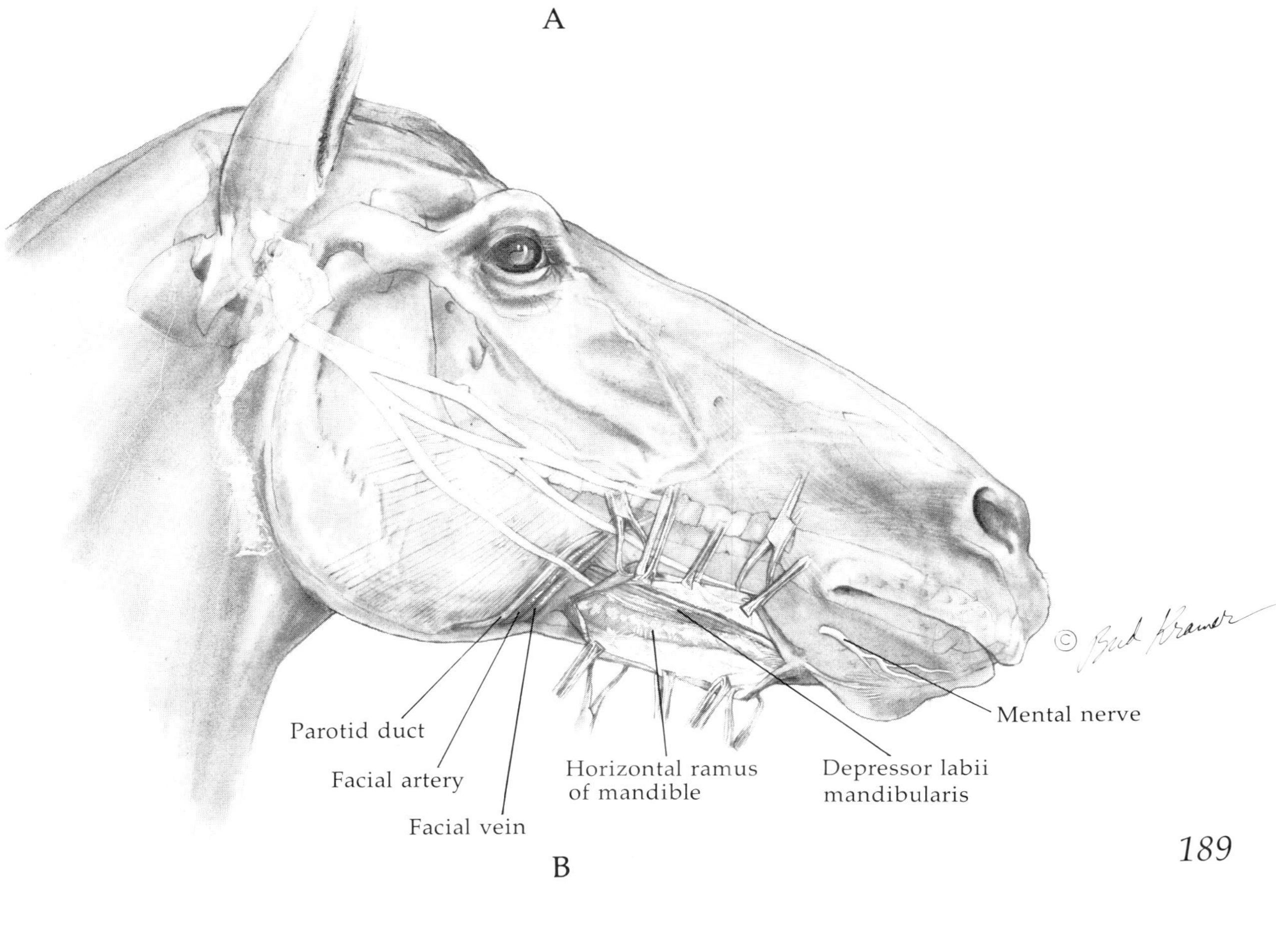

B

C. Surgeon's View. The depressor labii maxillaris muscle is reflected dorsally by elevating it from the lateral aspect of the horizontal ramus using a periosteal elevator. This exposes the lateral aspect of the horizontal ramus of the mandible.

CLOSURE

The subcutaneous fascia is closed using a continuous or interrupted suture pattern. The skin should be closed using an interrupted suture pattern so that the incised edges are in firm apposition.

LATERAL APPROACH TO THE HORIZONTAL RAMUS OF THE MANDIBLE

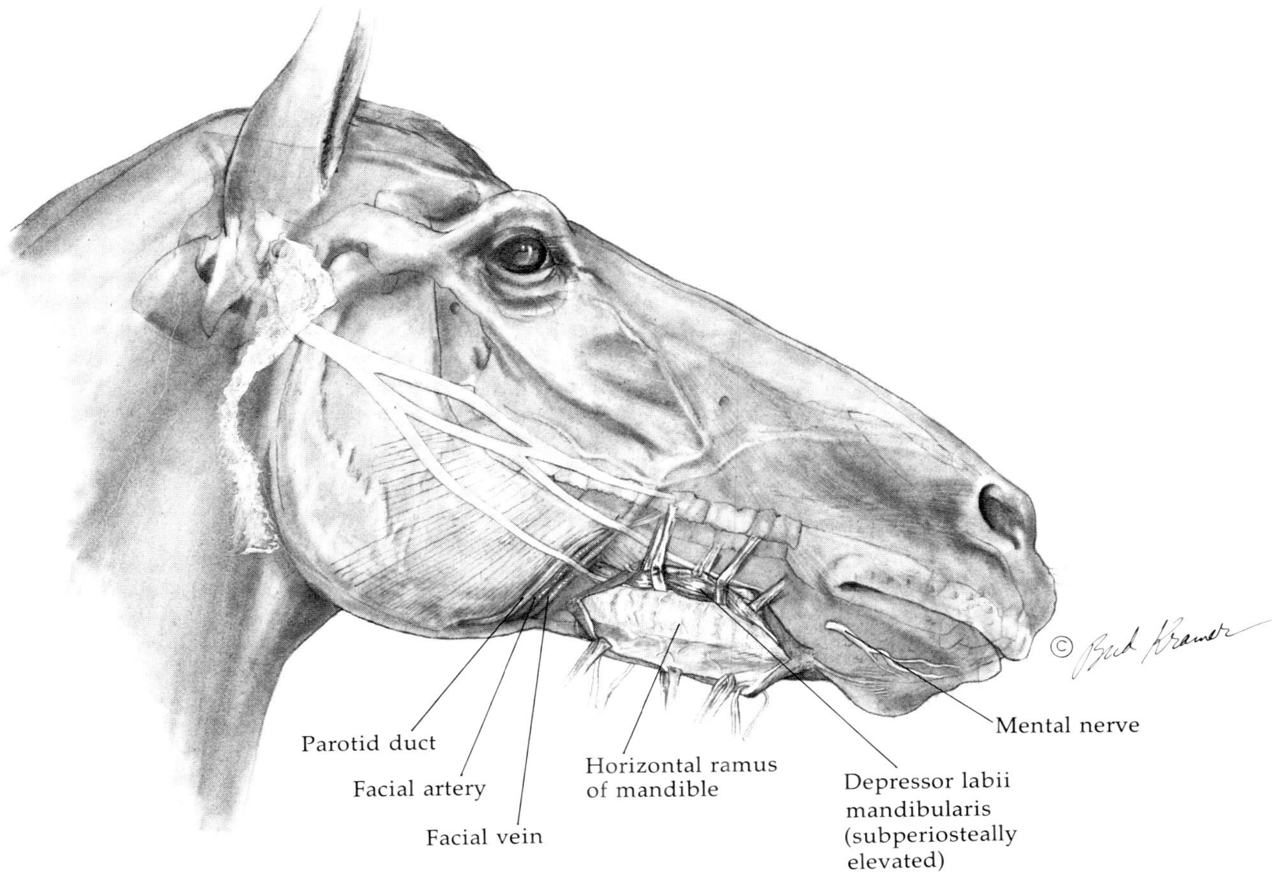

C

part four

Approach to the Lateral Aspect of the Maxilla and Incisive Bone

LATERAL APPROACH TO THE MAXILLA AND INCISIVE BONE (PREMAXILLA)

INDICATION

1. Open reduction and fixation of fractures of the maxilla and incisive bone.

POSITIONING OF PATIENT

The patient is placed with affected side uppermost.

DESCRIPTION OF PROCEDURE

A. Topographical View. A skin incision is made just dorsal and parallel to the tendon of the levator labii maxillaris muscle, extending from the nasoincisive notch to the level of the angular artery and vein of the eye.

B. Diagrammatic View Showing Muscles, Vessels and Nerves in Relationship to Bones. The angular artery and vein run toward the medial canthus of the eye along the caudal border of the levator nasolabialis muscle. The infraorbital nerve emerges from the infraorbital foramen medial to the levator labii maxillaris muscle. The lateral nasal artery and corresponding vein pass medial to the levator nasolabialis muscle and course along the ventral border of the levator labii maxillaris muscle. These vessels and nerves should be identified and preserved.

LATERAL APPROACH TO THE MAXILLA AND INCISIVE BONE (PREMAXILLA)

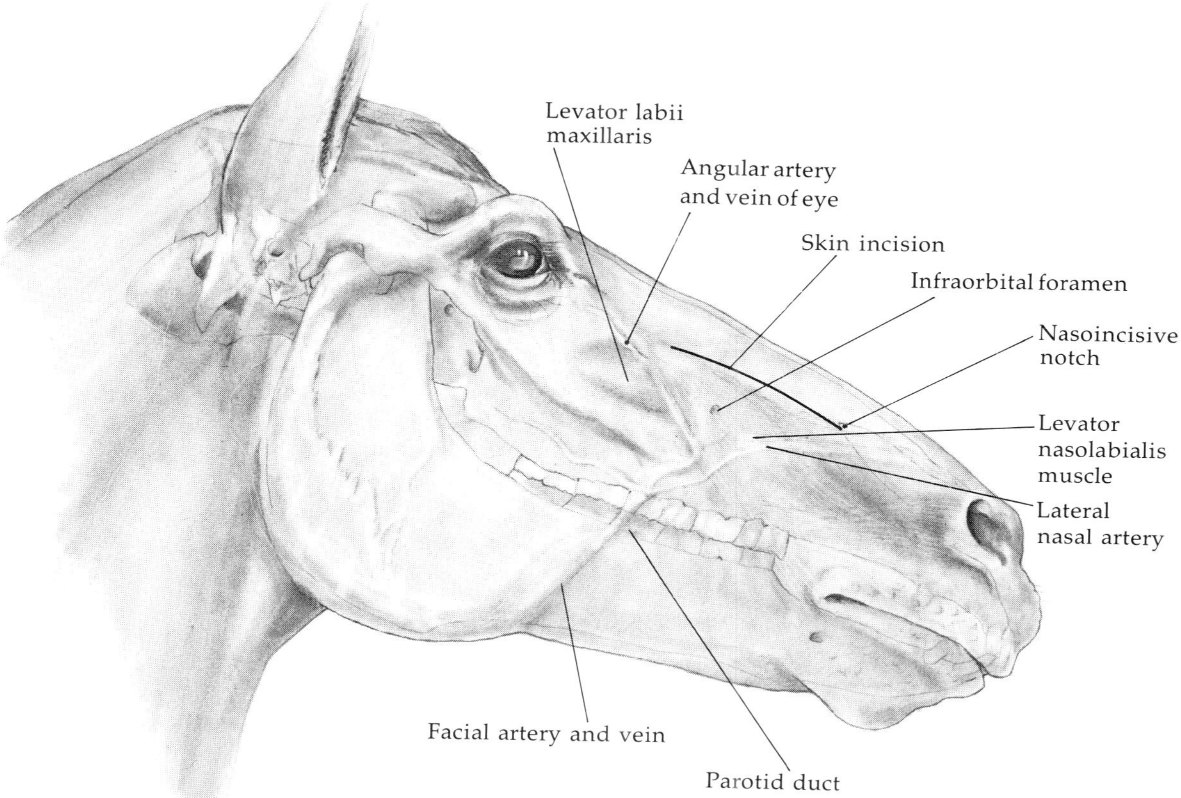

A

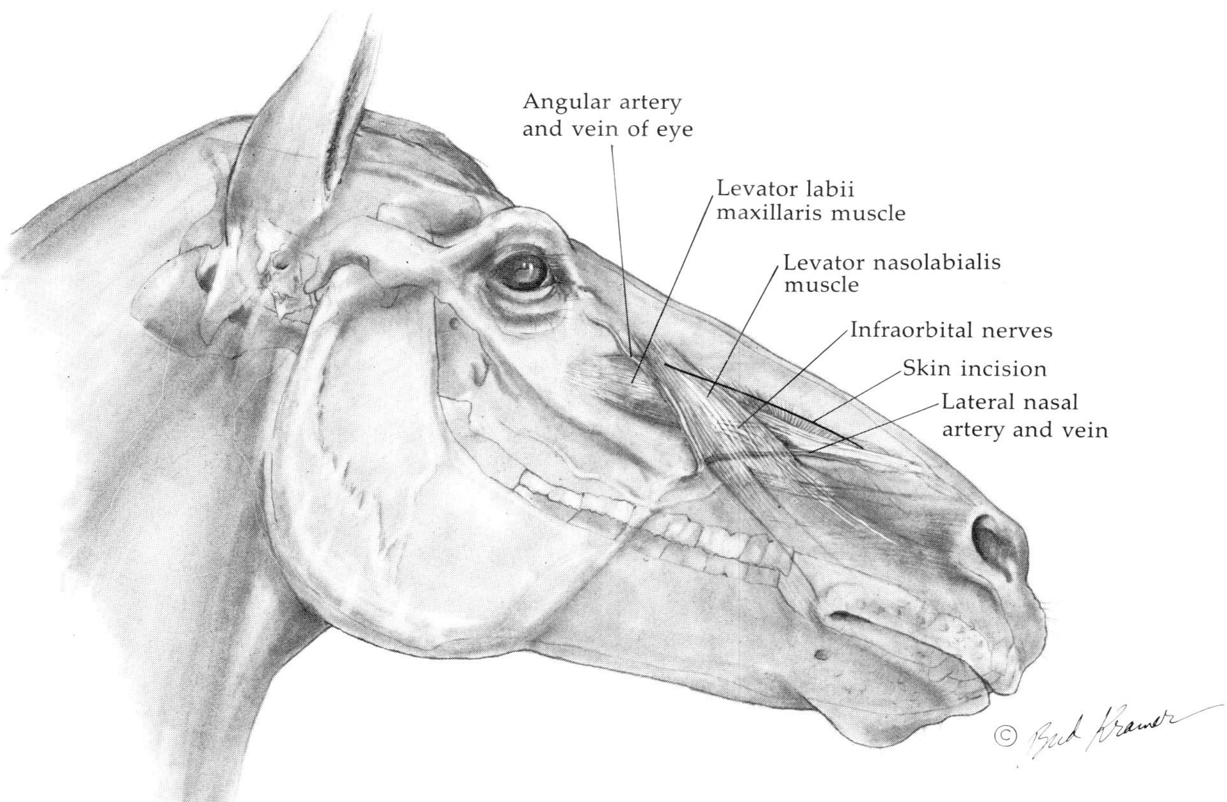

B

C. Surgeon's View. The subcutaneous fascia is incised along the same line as the skin incision. This exposes the levator nasolabialis muscle, which crosses the levator labii maxillaris muscle and tendon.

D. Surgeon's View. The levator nasolabialis is incised where it crosses the levator labii maxillaris. The two incised edges are reflected revealing the levator labii maxillaris muscle and tendon directly below. The levator labii maxillaris muscle and tendon are reflected ventrally, revealing the dorsal-lateral aspect of the maxilla and incisive bone. When reflecting this muscle belly, care should be taken to identify and preserve the infraorbital nerve (which emerges from the infraorbital foramen) and the lateral nasal artery.

CLOSURE

The levator nasolabialis muscle is closed with a simple interrupted pattern, the subcutaneous fascia is closed with a continuous interrupted pattern. The skin should be closed with an interrupted pattern so that the incised edges are in firm apposition.

COMMENTS

The approach only exposes the most caudal aspect of the incisive bone (premaxilla) and most rostral lateral aspect of the maxilla. The exposure is inadequate for visualization of the rostral-lateral aspect of the incisive bone; for exposure of this aspect of the incisive bone, the intraoral approach is used. Care must be taken not to enter the diverticulum (false nostril) with this approach.

Reference

1. Turner, A. S.: Surgical Management of Depression Fractures of the Equine Skull. J. Vet. Surg. (1979). (In press.)

LATERAL APPROACH TO THE MAXILLA AND INCISIVE BONE (PREMAXILLA)

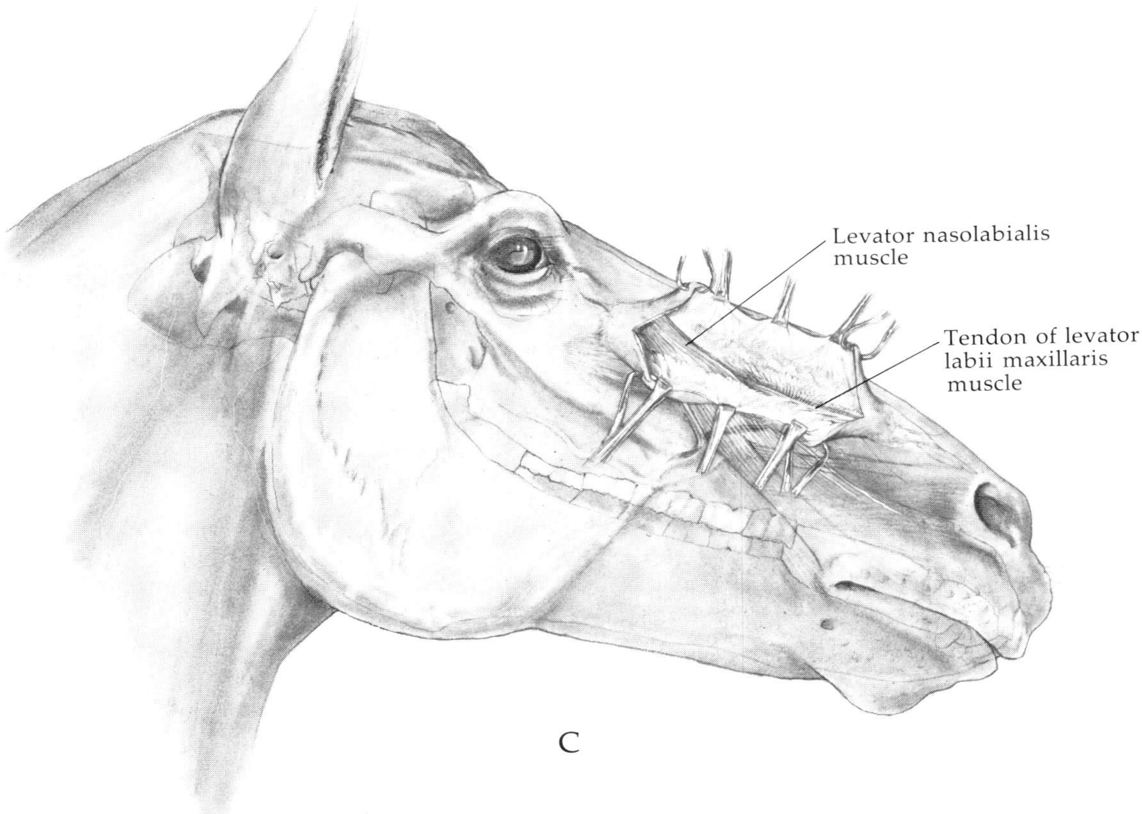

C

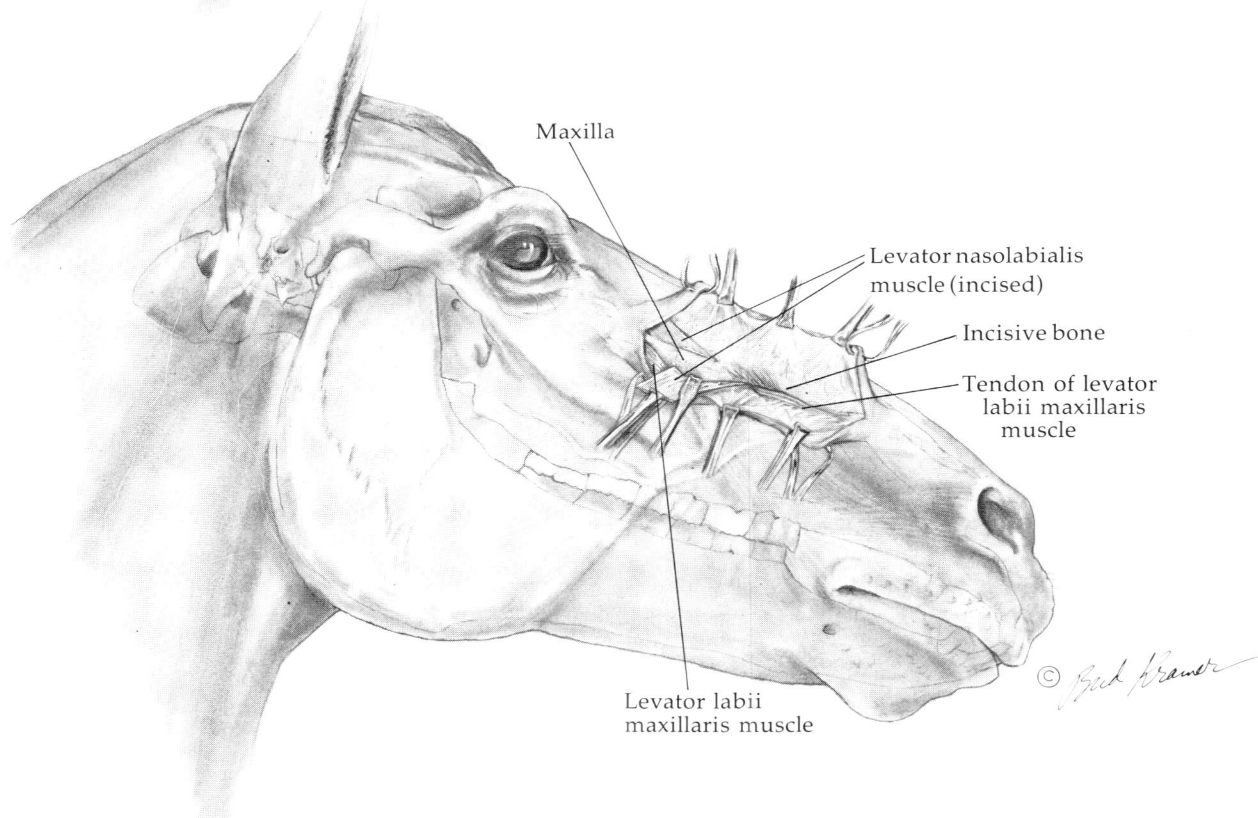

D

part five

Oral Approach to the Incisive Bone

ORAL APPROACH TO INCISIVE BONE

INDICATION

1. Open reduction and fixation of fractures of the body and nasal process of the incisive bone.

POSITIONING OF PATIENT

The patient is placed in dorsal recumbency with the ventral surface of the horizontal mandible pointing up. The mouth is held open with an appropriate mouth gag.

DESCRIPTION OF PROCEDURE

A. *Topographical View.* An incision approximately 4 cm. long is made through the gingiva down to and through the periosteum of the ventral aspect of the incisive bone. The incision extends from the first premolar to the corner incisor. The incision can be extended along the base of the center and middle incisor teeth if the body of incisive bone needs to be exposed.

B. *Surgeon's View.* The gingiva covering the ventral and lateral aspect of the incisive bone is subperiosteally elevated, exposing the ventral-lateral body and the nasal process of the incisive bone.

CLOSURE

The gingiva is closed using a simple interrupted suture pattern.

COMMENTS

This approach is used to expose the more rostral aspect of the incisive bone. The lateral approach is required to expose the caudal aspect.

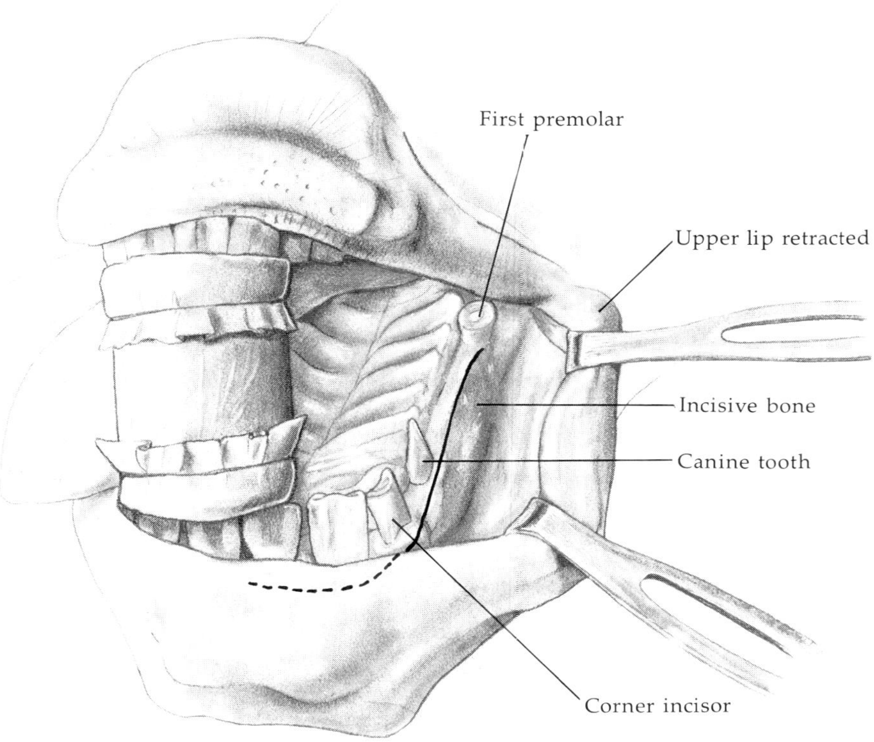
First premolar
Upper lip retracted
Incisive bone
Canine tooth
Corner incisor

A

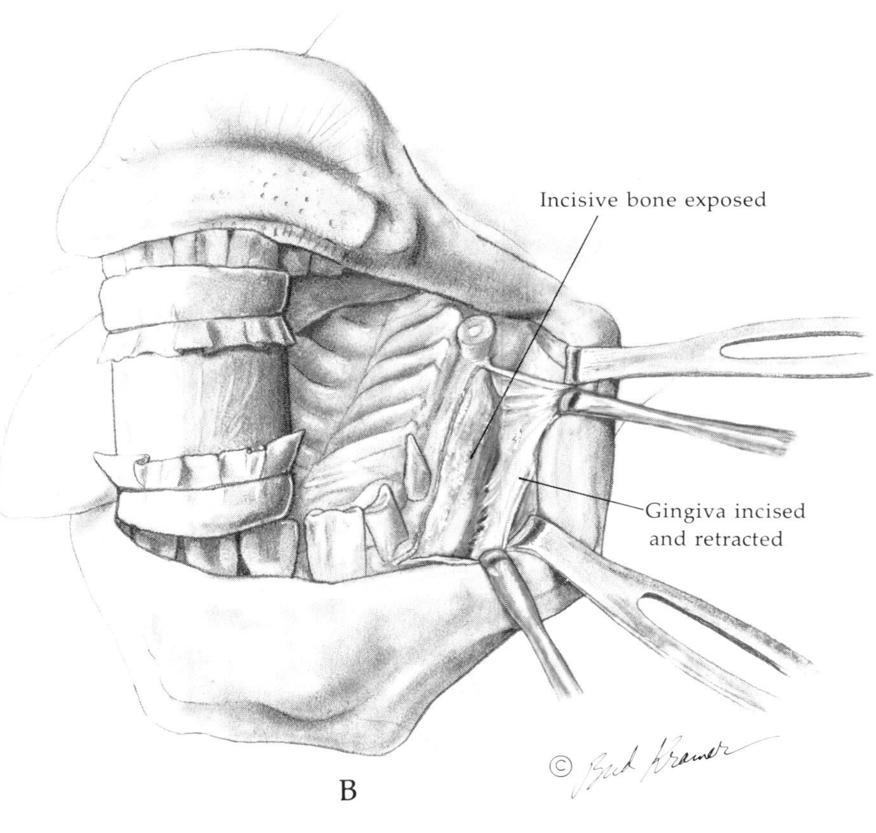
Incisive bone exposed
Gingiva incised
and retracted
© Bud Kramer

B

part six

Approach to the Frontal and Nasal Bones

APPROACH TO THE FRONTAL AND NASAL BONES

INDICATION

1. Open reduction and fixation of fracture of the frontal and nasal bones.[1–3]

POSITIONING OF PATIENT

The patient is positioned in lateral recumbency with the affected side uppermost.

DESCRIPTION OF PROCEDURE

A. *Topographical View.* A curvilinear skin incision approximately 20 cm. long is made from the level of the supraorbital foramen to the middle of the nasal process of the incisive bone. The apex of the incision is directed lateral to the midline of the forehead, to the right or left, depending on which direction provides the best exposure for the fracture presented.

B. *The Surgeon's View.* The skin is reflected from the subcutaneous fascia, exposing the underlying frontal and nasal bones.

CLOSURE

The skin should be closed using a simple interrupted suture pattern so that the incised edges are in firm apposition.

COMMENTS

The exact location of the skin incision will depend on the location of the fracture(s). The skin incision should be placed so that the flap area exposed extends beyond the margins of the fracture site. This will provide the surgeon with access to the surrounding stable, healthy bone for placement of wire sutures. It also provides freedom to choose strategic locations for small holes used to insert instruments sometimes needed to elevate depression fractures.[2]

References

1. Hertsch, B. R., Zeller, R., Wibdorf, H., and Hurtienne, H.: Contribution to the Treatment of Fractures of the Head of the Horse III. Fractures of the Facial Cranium. Dtsch. Tierarztl. Wschr. *83* (1976):263–314.
2. Turner, A. S.: Surgical Management of Depression Fractures of the Equine Skull. J. Vet. Surg. Vol. 8 (1979). (In press.)
3. Wheat, J. D.: Fractures of the Head and Mandible of the Horse. *In* Proceedings American Association of Equine Practitioners, 1975. (1976):223–228.

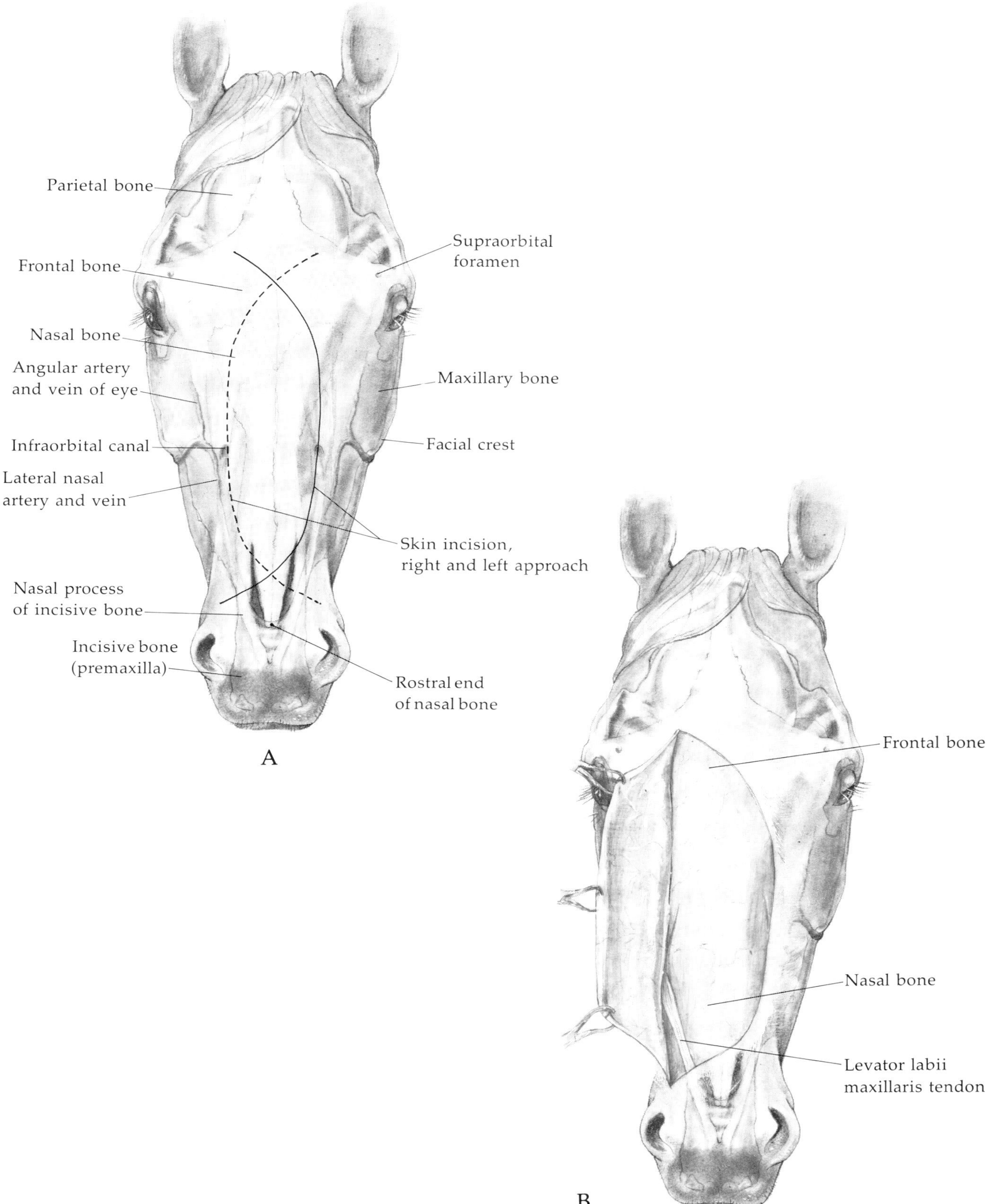
Parietal bone
Frontal bone
Nasal bone
Angular artery and vein of eye
Infraorbital canal
Lateral nasal artery and vein
Nasal process of incisive bone
Incisive bone (premaxilla)
Supraorbital foramen
Maxillary bone
Facial crest
Skin incision, right and left approach
Rostral end of nasal bone
A
Frontal bone
Nasal bone
Levator labii maxillaris tendon
B

Index

Note: Page numbers in *italics* refer to illustrations.